NORMAN CAMPBELL is a man of humble origins who struggled to finance his own education, eventually succeeding in obtaining an MSc in Mathematics. During his final year at university, he was struck down by schizophrenia, only making a good recovery in later life as a result of his Christian convictions and modern medication.

How I Defeated Schizophrenia

How I Defeated Schizophrenia

Norman Campbell

ATHENA PRESS
LONDON

ISBN 978 1 84748 584 7

First published 2009 by
ATHENA PRESS
Queen's House, 2 Holly Road
Twickenham TW1 4EG
United Kingdom

Printed for Athena Press

A Brief Introduction

I wrote this book to illustrate how, if one perseveres, one can overcome mental illness. I have drawn a comparison between my past mental state and my present one. References have been made to factors that influenced my decline into schizophrenia and those that influenced my recovery. I have stressed the importance of my Christian faith to me, and am convinced that we all have to face judgement one day. I certainly need forgiveness for my immoral past and I have repented of the behaviour I was involved in. I feel that I am better able to come to terms now with these sad episodes in my past through my Christian faith and the certainty of forgiveness by God. I hope that my book will serve as an inspiration to those who have faced the same problems that I have encountered.

Contents

Chapter One – Beginnings

Bayble was an island community of about eighty dwellings situated a mile from a picturesque bay off the north-west coast of Scotland, and it was here that Norman spent his youth. A good view of the bay was afforded from one of the windows of his dwelling, and the unpredictability of the weather was easily apparent due to the fact that an indication of how stormy it was at any particular time was the height of the breaking waves over a sea stack in the distance. The weather could change rapidly from one extreme to another. There was no such variation in the general religious conviction of the villagers, for whom the acknowledgement of God as a stable guiding influence in their lives was always exhibited through their regular churchgoing and adherence to Calvinistic doctrine.

A person's mood can usually be influenced by the weather, which comes with the changing seasons; but it did not influence the adult members of the Bayble community, who had become hardened to the fickleness of the weather. The children, however, were filled with wonder at the white snowy expanses of winter-time; Norman was no exception, and as a child he was fascinated by the descent of the snowflakes from the skies – their source unexplainable – fluttering gently to the ground and covering it with a carpet of white as far as the eye could see. Children can be very impressionable, and their experiences at an early age can have a pronounced effect on how their character can be moulded. While Norman grew up with his mother, his father and mother were never together, due to the simple fact that his father was married to someone else.

Life was idyllic for him as a child, up to the point when he discovered, through his companions, that everybody had a father. He had been of the opinion that his father had never existed, but this was a rude awakening to him. An incident at school a year previously came to his mind and he remembered a discussion he had had with a fellow pupil called Hector.

'I hear your father is a doctor, Hector.'

'What does your father do, Norman?'

Norman replied innocently, 'I have no father.'

Hector's reaction was one of disbelief and he stated firmly, 'We all have fathers, Norman, and you are no exception.'

A pupil who had overheard the conversation started sniggering, a reaction which Norman found puzzling and unexplainable at the time but which could now be clarified in the light of his recent understanding of the inevitability of there being a father for all of us. Later in life, having committed his life to Jesus and his Father in heaven, Norman would be comforted by the Scriptures in regard to the absence of a human father:

> If anyone comes to me and does not hate his father and his mother, his wife and children – yes, even his own life – he cannot be my disciple.

The absence of a father to give Norman guidance and advice in his teenage years would prove to be a problem for him. He found it difficult to communicate with his mother when he encountered setbacks in life. There was something incomplete about his family relationship that would become more pronounced as time went on.

Sexual awakening can prompt a child to ask questions about procreation, and Norman was no exception. However, the sordid details about the absence of a father and the fact that his father's identity had never been intimated to him tainted his view of sexual relations. The word used as a swear word to denote someone who was illegitimate was often bandied about by children, and every time it was used in Norman's presence he felt it was levelled at himself. He tried to summon up the courage to approach his mother and ask her to reveal his father's identity, but since his mother had remained silent about that topic for thirteen years Norman sensed that she would find that sort of discussion distasteful; so he postponed it, and never actually asked for an explanation. Her decision not to discuss his father's identity was perfectly understandable, as it would have probably caused her deep embarrassment and pain. However, she was to bring him up with love and care despite the incompleteness of the family unit.

Shortly afterwards, Norman experienced sharp pains in his groin. He was unable to confide in anyone due to the location of the pains and reduced his physical activities to a minimum. Eventually his toes developed a bluish colour, and this he was able to reveal to his mother.

'I think you are suffering from an abscess and I have decided to treat it by applying poultices to the affected sites.'

She proceeded to implement this decision, Norman finding the heat a trifle unbearable. He protested. 'Is it absolutely necessary to proceed towards a cure using that method?'

'Yes. I am confident it will work, and will say a prayer to God asking Him to intercede and heal you. I suggest you confine yourself to bed until you recover.'

Being an obedient child, and hoping that a rest in bed would be the solution to his pains and other symptoms, he submitted to his mother's authority and spent the next day or two in bed. The discomfort of the straw mattress diverted his thoughts from the area affected by the pain to other areas of his body which were in contact with the protruding parts of the mattress.

Next day his mother inspected his toes, and seeing that there was no improvement, she said, 'It looks more serious than I anticipated, and I fear that it will be necessary to telephone the doctor to come and visit you. You are probably aware that he will have to make a seven-mile journey to get here, but I do think it is essential that we seek proper medical aid under the circumstances. Try not to worry. I am strongly of the opinion that this decision is the right one.'

Immediately she donned a coat and proceeded to walk to the nearest telephone kiosk, which was half a mile distant. The coat she had hastily covered herself with was to protect her from the rain, which seemed inevitable judging by the dark and ominous clouds. It was summer, but the area was susceptible to heavy showers which could materialise unexpectedly at any moment. She showed her concern for her son's predicament by the transformation of her walk to a faster lope. Soon the weather deteriorated and the rain came down in torrents. Despite the downpour she never faltered, and eventually she arrived at the telephone kiosk, from which she was able to extract a promise from the doctor to come as soon as possible. Having completed her journey successfully, she breathed a sigh of relief and headed back home, the rain having abated. She was confident about the outcome because she put the matter in God's hands and felt that her faith would see her through her son's misfortune. She arrived home and they both waited expectantly for the doctor to arrive.

The sun had by now dispelled the clouds, and the numerous and varying flowers which carpeted the ground could vie in beauty with the most attractive of Matisse's patterned backgrounds. Unfortunately they wither and perish within a short space of time and are indicative of 'life's little day', if one pauses to reflect on those matters. Norman was not reflecting on the distant future but was preoccupied with the present and the short-term future, which he hoped would involve the opposite sex. He had reached the stage in life where these thoughts dominated. He would often be able to suppress unpleasant thoughts by focusing on fantasies involving girls. This was his mood when the doctor made his appearance an hour later. The doctor started his examination of Norman's discoloured toes and asked him in a gentle and fatherly tone (fatherly probably because he knew Norman had lacked a father up to that point), 'Do you have any pain anywhere?'

Norman's first reaction was to respond in the negative but he found the doctor's tone reassuring, and summoning up his courage he replied, 'I have pain here.'

Norman indicated the site of the pain.

'I am going to take your temperature. Hold still while I insert the thermometer under your tongue. A thermometer indicates the body temperature and this is useful in making a diagnosis. You have probably encountered thermometers in your physics class at school.'

After a few seconds had elapsed he withdrew the thermometer and looked at the reading. He did not hesitate, and confided in Nora, Norman's mother, 'He has contacted rheumatic fever and will have to be admitted to the local hospital immediately. He will be treated there by medical staff; this is essential to his recovery rather than undergoing his treatment at home. I have not detected any abnormality with his heart at this stage, and hopefully after a period of rest in hospital he will make a good recovery. I have decided he should be admitted today and will phone for an ambulance to collect him. You should make all necessary preparations in the meantime for his stay at hospital.'

Nora replied, 'I am grateful to you, Doctor. I regret I didn't make an accurate assessment of my son's illness and summon you yesterday. Thank you for your assistance.'

Whenever Norman looked back on these events when he was much older, they seemed hazy and uncertain. When he would develop schizophrenia he would look back to this examination by the doctor in a way that didn't reflect the truth. He would see himself in the bed exhibiting stupor – a symptom of catatonic schizophrenia. The memory, possibly false, would remain vividly embedded in his mind and would never be erased.

The doctor then departed on his journey back to his surgery, which was located in the town seven miles away. Despite the doctor's reassurance, Nora had become anxious at the way the situation had developed and was concerned in case her delay in contacting the doctor might have possibly serious repercussions. Then she comforted herself with the thought that Jesus had healed a blind man by applying mud to his eyes and asking him to wash them in the pool of Siloam. Her application of poultices to the affected toes had reminded her of that miracle, and she recovered her composure and packed a little case with all the items Norman would need during his stay at the hospital.

Eventually the ambulance arrived, and Norman was conveyed on a stretcher into the ambulance – without his mother to accompany him as she had to care for his sister and grandparents. 'Take up your mat and walk' was not applicable at that particular time, but Nora was convinced that it would be relevant in the fullness of time. He was carried on the stretcher into the adult ward of the hospital, as it was deemed more suitable than a children's ward due to Norman being thirteen years of age. The medical staff felt he would be more settled among adults. A nurse took down his details while he lay on the stretcher, before he was actually admitted to the ward. A young, inexperienced nurse tried to extract all the information she required from Norman and started with the question, 'What is your father's name?'

This was an embarrassing question for him as he had recently discovered that he was born out of wedlock. His father's surname would be expected to be the same as his own, so he supplied his grandfather's name instead and said, 'My father's name is Donald Campbell.'

Immediately he felt a sense of embarrassment at this false admission. He had already begun to associate paternity with shame and embarrassment. His pressing thought as he was transferred from the stretcher to the bed was the fear that his lie would be discovered. His mood became agitated as the nurse continued with her questions, and he breathed a sigh of relief as she concluded her inquiries, saving him the discomfort of having to resort to more lies. The fact that his interrogator was female made the situation more awkward, as he felt she would despise him for being illegitimate. Due to the emptiness in his life, which he felt from not having a father present, and the way in which he had discovered it, he was beginning to associate sex with shame. He pondered over the identity of his actual father, and the foolish thought came into his mind that he had provided the nurse with the right answer to her first question. The thought was disturbing and would return to haunt him later in life.

He was cared for over a long period, with complete rest accompanying his medical treatment. It was essential that he remain confined to bed for several months to prevent his heart from being affected by the rheumatic fever. It was known to cause problems with the heart valves and this could result in serious complications. Aspirin was administered in quite large quantities at the beginning of the treatment. The nurses were very attentive and Norman found the nurse who had questioned him prior to his admission more appealing than the others. On one occasion she manicured his fingernails and drew attention to the cuticles. 'They are called cuticles. Do you know what the word "cute" means? You sometimes apply that adjective to people that you like a lot. Who would you describe as cute, Norman?'

'I think I would describe you in those terms,' he retorted. He sensed that she was endeavouring to steer the conversation in a certain direction and waited for her reaction to his statement.

She thought for a while and hesitated before replying gently, 'I find Dr Reid very cute, but promise me you won't tell anyone… There are other people I adore too but I find him the cutest. I love his bedside manner and his compassion for those who are suffering here. Do you think he might find me cute too?'

'I did notice he seemed to show some affection to you. I don't know if he thinks you're cute but I have a confession to make: I like you a lot. Call me a fool, but I felt I had to reveal my feelings to you.'

'Norman, I do have a high regard for you, but as I have stated I have lost my heart to Dr Reid. I am certain that when you recover and depart from hospital you will find a sweet female companion to be at your side instead of me.'

Having said this she departed and left Norman to collect his thoughts. He felt disappointed she had admitted that she admired Dr Reid, but had some consolation from her flattering comment about himself, which she had the grace to make. However, he had to admit to himself that he would love to be Dr Reid, and from that moment onwards he admired doctors in general.

He felt very conscious of the fact that he had no pyjamas on and had to leave his shirt on to cover his nakedness. On his mother's first visit she provided him with one she had specially bought, out of her poverty. It all served to remind Norman that his family was different from many others and was perhaps the poorest in the village. There was no father to bring in a steady flow of money. His family depended totally on benefits. He became aware at this time that it was a father's duty to provide for his wife and children. However, the care bestowed on him by his mother, and her regular visits, served to strengthen the bond between them.

Three months had elapsed, and it was time Norman left his bed in which he had rested for such a long period. When he got on his feet he found he had to rely on the support of two nurses, one on either side, as his muscles had weakened due to the long period of inactivity. They reassured him that he would recover his strength before long, and they were right, as it happened. His mother had been visiting him regularly and was pleased with how he had progressed. She had often expressed her love for him on her visits and frequently brought him fruit and other food when visiting, despite being very poor. It was with a rush of realisation on one of those visits that Norman felt closer to her than he had ever been before. Caravaggio's 'Supper at Emmaus' seems appropriate at this time, depicting the scene when the two disciples realise that their companion is in fact Jesus himself.

'Whoever visits my sick does it for me...'

He sensed then that she was someone precious to him. On his last day at hospital, during his departure he received the good wishes of the hospital staff and was escorted to an ambulance which conveyed him home.

Having become aware of procreation and all that was connected with it, Norman's views on these topics were to undergo a change. It seemed to him that there was no obstacle to sexual intercourse if contraceptives were found. It seemed to him the only hurdle to be faced for success in that area. Even these precautions might be dispensed with, he thought. However, the subject of sex was tinged with embarrassment for him, due to his own family situation. He found out quite quickly that girls were not an easy proposition – those around him in particular, as religious beliefs were quite strong in that part of the world. Although premarital sex occurred there, it was deeply frowned on and families in his situation gained the disapproval of the Church. 'Neighbours here we can love' – but obviously not in the carnal sense, would be the Church's stance. He confided in a friend called Donald about his feelings but did not find a solution to his problem there. On one occasion in Donald's home he intimated to him, 'I am puzzled about the identity of my father. Maybe I should call him Mr X, the unknown. I have no ideas who he is. Every man about my mother's age is a candidate, owing due to my uncertainty about his identity.'

'Wait here a moment until I consult my mother in the next room,' Donald replied.

He returned after a short delay of a few minutes and asked, 'You know your cousin Rosie in London? Well, she could be your close relative.'

'I fail to understand your implication, Donald, and don't think you have answered my question properly. I cannot understand why my mother never brought the subject up. I suppose I shall have to remain ignorant until she chooses to bring the topic up. I do feel there has been a vacuum created in my life since I discovered we all possess a father.'

Several months afterwards, Norman happened to be sitting at a table at home and was oblivious to the fact that he was moving about in a restless way. Nora, his mother, happened to notice that he kept shifting his position and asked him to try and control his restlessness. Norman was unable to comply, and next morning Nora supplied him with a note for his doctor, who was asked in the note to investigate his uncontrolled movements. The doctor had his surgery in town and Norman duly visited him after school. On entering the doctor's surgery, Norman gave the note to the doctor, who said, 'Remove your braces so that I can examine your heart with my stethoscope. There is nothing to worry about.'

Norman attempted to remove his braces, but his jerking movements resulted in his buttons tearing and his embarrassment was intensified by the look of concern on the doctor's face. When he had completed his examination he said, 'I will write a letter to your mother with instructions about what to do. Make sure you deliver it to her.'

He had made the diagnosis of rheumatic chorea, and had requested Norman's mother to convey him urgently to hospital, which she did.

On arrival to hospital he was admitted to a private room, as they felt he could be better managed there. He was unaware of the reason why he had been taken into hospital and asked a nurse what the nature of his illness was. He felt relieved when she clarified the situation to him, as he had felt bewildered and confused about what was happening to him. He asked about his favourite nurse, who had tended him during his admittance with rheumatic fever, but to his disappointment he was told she had left and was no longer working there. However he made eye contact with a blue-eyed nurse, who quickly replaced the previous nurse in Norman's affection. There was something about her gentle but purposeful movements that Norman found irresistibly attractive to him. Her body was full and curvaceous, and this heightened his desire for her. However his lack of control of his movements caused him acute embarrassment and created a severe problem with his relationships with other patients there, as he sensed they might attribute his uncontrolled movements to mental problems.

He remained an inpatient again for about three months. During this stay he met and made friends with a middle-aged teacher who was a patient there. The teacher probably looked on Norman as a pupil he could relate to and was quick to test Norman's intellectual ability. He gave him a list of Scottish towns and associated products for which they were famous for manufacturing, and said, 'Memorise as much of the details on the list as you can for five minutes, and afterwards I will test you to see how many you remember.'

After the five minutes had elapsed the teacher received the list back and said, 'I will announce each town in turn and you supply the associated product relating to each town.'

He was very impressed by the fact that Norman had memorised everything with the exception of a couple of towns, and stated that he thought Norman was very intelligent.

'I have a secret to confide in you,' Norman told him. 'I am illegitimate, and feel that the opposite sex find that distasteful. Do not reveal this to any of the nurses, as I am very fond of some of them and don't wish to lose their affection. Intelligence doesn't mean so much to me as the constancy of their affection. Have you any knowledge of how women feel towards people like me?'

The answer given did not satisfy Norman, who regretted having brought the subject up in the first place. It was a mistake, he thought, and it made him more vulnerable now during the rest of his stay in hospital. He had thought that taking the teacher into his confidence would ease his feeling of embarrassment, but this was not the case. In due course Norman was discharged and returned home.

The poverty of his family's existence was emphasised during Norman's first meal on coming back home. It was a simple meal of herring and potatoes, which Norman insisted eating with a knife and fork. He had become accustomed to using cutlery in hospital and his grandfather remarked that Norman was behaving in a superior way. This difference in lifestyle made him feel even more isolated from his wealthier neighbours. There was now an emptiness in his life which took some time to dissipate, as he had revelled in the nurses' kindness at hospital. There was no substitute for this, as he had no close female relationships to fall back on outside hospital. He had now to resume his career at school, having lost a year due to his two absences. Gradually his memory of his hospital admissions faded a bit, but he was acutely aware that his companions might view his second illness as suggestive of mental derangement.

Chapter Two – Restarting School

Norman had to resume his schooling in the autumn. Since he had been absent for over a year due to his illnesses and recuperation, he had to restart with the class that had been below his in the past. Being unfamiliar with the pupils in that class, he had to forge new relationships, and with a conscious determination he set about this. He introduced himself to the others at the first opportunity, which was after school diner in the cloakroom. He approached one fellow pupil and said, 'My name is Norman. A year has elapsed since the time I first became ill with rheumatic fever. As a result of this I have had to be placed in the class that used to be below me. The absence wasn't really that long and amounted to a prolonged holiday for me. To be honest I didn't miss it.'

The other pupil replied, 'I'm Corrie. I gather that you had another illness, which I am curious about, connected to the rheumatic fever. Can you describe it?'

'Yes,' replied Norman, 'Its main feature is the loss of control over one's movements, which are executed in a jerky manner. I remember being in the hospital bed soon after being admitted, reaching for a glass of water on the bedside cabinet, picking it up without proper control, with the result that it dropped out of my hand on to the floor, where it completely fragmented. A nurse soon appeared at my bedside and suggested I call her if I needed anything, even the most insignificant thing. I felt responsible for the accident but she was very understanding. The medical name for the illness is rheumatic chorea, but it is also known as St Vitus's dance.'

Norman had to summon up all his courage to supply the latter name as to him it seemed to suggest a deliberate and conscious behaviour of a bizarre type. Corrie was quite interested in the description, to which he listened without interruption. Norman felt he was more understanding than the other pupils, who were talking animatedly among themselves in various groups. However, he had an uneasy and disturbing feeling that the others were discussing his illness, as Corrie had brought the subject up.

'Thanks for your explanation, Norman,' Corrie retorted, 'I hope you are successful in becoming integrated into the class over the next few months.'

As it transpired, no one else questioned Norman about the illness he had suffered from and he felt concerned in case they might have found the topic too delicate to discuss. He needed someone to materialise out of thin air and greet him with the words, 'Peace be with you'. Although physically close to the other children, he felt worlds separated him from them in social interaction and he felt very isolated and alone in that particular situation. Having recently experienced sexual awakening, he was also conscious now that there was a stigma attached to illegitimacy, and he preferred to hope that his family situation had not become known to the others in his school. There were one or two others from the same village as his at the school and he felt that they might have revealed all. He really felt that there was something inferior about himself as a person, mainly due to the common usage of the word 'bastard', which was used as a term of belittlement. Every time he heard that word being used he felt it was directed at him, and that added more fuel to the destructive fire that was burning inside him. After school he would return to his country village where all were aware of the background of his family.

It seemed to him as if he was living in two distinct worlds – here in one world they knew, in the other perhaps they didn't. During the dinner break and after the school dinner the pupils would gather in the cloakroom to talk until they were summoned back to class by the school bell. Norman did not take part in the exchanges and felt that the banter and laughter of the others were directed at him. He felt an acute feeling of persecution and tried to occupy himself by reading a newspaper while the others talked among themselves. Their laughter was almost unbearable to him.

He had few female contacts with whom he could relate. While waiting for a bus to convey him home from school one evening, he happened to have a conversation with a girl about his own age who resided locally in the town.

'I haven't seen you around this area before. My name is Joan,' she said.

He tried not to display any indication that he had noticed her developing bust, and although it was far from being fully developed there was something about its very existence that he found so very appealing. He fixed his eyes on her and tried not to betray his real thoughts – that he was attracted physically to her.

'My name is Norman,' was his reply. 'I chanced to be here at this particular time as I have missed my bus home and will have to wait for the next one, which is due in an hour's time.'

'There is a dance taking place in the town hall this evening and I haven't got a partner,' she said. 'Would you like to accompany me?'

Norman was unable to accept the invitation as he had to admit that he couldn't dance. He felt flattered by her approach. The way the males were segregated from the females during school hours had made intersexual relations quite difficult during that period, and his inability to mix with girls socially only served to increase his feelings of inadequacy. The response of feeling sexually attracted to females was accompanied simultaneously by a feeling that sexual feelings were shameful. This made barriers between the two sexes difficult to break down, but Joan had succeeded where others might have failed. Her boldness captivated him.

'I like you more than anyone I have ever met before and would like to continue our relationship by meeting you here regularly after school,' he said courageously, hoping that she would respond positively. She smiled at him warmly with a favourable reaction.

'There was something about you which attracted me to you, definitely not the fact that you were the only male around these parts. What do you like best about me?' she asked petulantly.

Norman gazed at her face appreciatively and their eyes met and interlocked for what seemed to be an eternity. He avoided looking at her from head to toe, although this is what he instinctively felt like doing, and his imagination ran free because what he saw was the Venus shaped by Bronzino in his erotic 'Allegory of Venus and Cupid'.

'I find your brown eyes very desirable,' he said, evading a truthful answer.

He exacted a promise from her that they should meet again at the same spot, and after a long conversation during which they exchanged information about themselves they parted company on the arrival of Norman's bus. On the half-hour journey home in the bus Norman felt a feeling of elation which nothing could dispel, as his mind ran over the preceding events. He did not share his experience with anyone and hoped that his relationship with the girl would eventually blossom into a physical one. That was the dominant feeling he had about their relationship; his mind was full of the most intimate details on that score. He would soon have his hopes dashed – and rightly so, for human relationships should be built on the right kind of love. The quote from the Gospels – 'Whoever looks at a woman lustfully has already committed adultery with her in his heart' – certainly applied to Norman as he let his imagination run riot afterwards.

Next evening Norman waited expectantly at the bus parking area for Joan to appear again. The location where they choose to meet was hardly conducive to romance, as a strong smell of salted herring pervaded the air. One of Norman's neighbours had been employed to salt herrings near that area. They were placed in a barrel in layers with salt sprinkled over each layer until the barrel was filled. Protective gloves were required in order to avoid prolonged contact with salt. A strong, unpleasant smell emanated from the herring, making him feel uneasy about the intended rendezvous. His eyes met the neighbour's and he acknowledged her presence by nodding, but she failed to respond and continued her labours with what seemed to him renewed vigour.

The sky had darkened and night would soon be approaching; Norman had a feeling of apprehension as he stood there waiting. The weather was unpredictable in that part of the country, and he resolved to find shelter from the likely downpour by sheltering in an empty bus, which would remain unattended until it was due to depart at a later time. The fact that the bus had been left unattended was an indication of the trust people placed in each other, crime there being virtually unheard of. In Norman's village house doors were never locked, even when its usual occupants were not present inside. Visitors just walked straight in.

The passage of time seemed to last an eternity, until he

noticed a group of young girls approaching, Joan being included in the group. They walked in his direction and when they reached him Joan introduced her companions, one of them apparently known as Hannah. She was wearing a leather coat, which he found appealing due to the fact that it clung to her body and made her appear very seductive.

'This is Hannah,' Joan continued, 'she is several years older than me but she's still unattached. We are all seeking male friends as there is a shortage of nice males where we come from.'

Norman had found Hannah even more seductive than Joan. Joan had been in his thoughts constantly since the previous day, but he decided not to reveal his feelings and addressed her. 'You are all very attractive. It was nice of you to bring your friends with you to meet me. I don't have many friends, unlike you.' He was taken aback by their forthright conversation and felt as if his inhibitions were melting away.

'I discussed the coming dance with Norman yesterday,' Joan replied, 'but he is reluctant to accompany me as he claims he cannot dance. Hannah and I will demonstrate the waltz. Observe us closely, Norman.'

They danced a few steps, and instead of inspiring Norman to attempt it himself, their performance made him more aware of his own shortcomings and he declined Joan's offer again. Although he responded to their banter, he was conscious all the time of the attraction their physical bodies had for him, and the object of the conversation seemed to him to be directed more to an intimate knowledge of their bodies rather than their minds.

At that moment it started to rain, and his female companions agreed to his suggestion that they should resume their conversation inside the empty bus. The pitter-patter of the raindrops echoed inside the bus and they all paused to listen to it as if it was an extension of their previous conversation.

'Who is your favourite singer?' Joan said, hoping that their musical tastes corresponded.

There was a pause on Norman's part and, after some reflection, he ventured to admit that it was Elvis Presley. The conversation had switched to pop music, with which he was quite familiar, so he endeavoured to focus as much of it as possible on this topic.

'Yes, he is mine as well,' she responded, 'I just love his latest song.'

That happened to be 'Heartbreak Hotel', and he knew it well, so he decided to discuss the lyrics. 'The conclusion of the song is rather sad,' he said. 'I would hate to undergo such suffering due to a breakdown in male–female relations. I hope it never happens to me.'

There was a dispute between them all as to whether Pat Boone was more charismatic than Elvis, but the general consensus was that Elvis reigned supreme.

'I admire Pat for his admission that he is a Christian,' Joan intervened, 'and he is very much respected by young and adults alike.'

Norman decided not to comment on this statement as he felt alienated by the latter singer's confession that he was a Christian. Norman's experience of church was a negative one, as he had problems learning his catechism, which was in Gaelic in Sunday school. He had never learnt how to read that language, although he was able to read English. Norman would come to believe at a future time that 'Let your light shine' was the right approach to life. The church elder who took his Sunday class happened to reveal that he was a cousin of Norman and was particularly understanding about Norman's struggle with reading Gaelic. There was something paternal about him that appealed to Norman.

After they'd sheltered in the bus for some time, a young girl called Christina entered and sat down beside them. She was rather an aggressive sort of girl but he had always admired her for her striking looks. For some inexplicable reason she suddenly shouted at his companions, 'Get out of the bus! Leave him alone! You are nothing but a bunch of whores.'

Her determination was such that she succeeded in her aim. His companions had asked him for his support but he had been unable to give it. He felt unable to understand her motive for her behaviour, and eventually he was alone in the empty bus. He somehow felt that he deserved what had come to pass due to his guilty feelings about his own attraction for the opposite sex. His female friends had deserted him and he was puzzled at how speedily they had done so. It seemed to him that they had been waiting for an event like that to happen, as their departure had been so sudden. He sat there bewildered, and did not accompany them out of the bus. A few moments later Christina returned and confronted him.

'You are a bastard!' said she. 'They were just making fun of you,' she continued derisively.

Norman felt the tears come to his eyes and immediately a flood of bitter, salty tears flooded down his face, almost drenching him like rain. She had destroyed the hope he had of developing a deeper relationship with Joan, and made him feel inadequate and inferior in the eyes of his companions. He remained mute and unresponsive to her criticisms and the tears kept flowing. His impression was that Christina thought him unworthy of maintaining the fragile relationship which had come to pass between him and Joan. When Christina observed the tears running down his face her demeanour changed and a shocked expression came to her face when she realised how much her verbal abuse had hurt his feelings. She withdrew and left Norman alone with his thoughts. He hated having revealed his feelings openly more than her actual words. Showing an emotional response openly was difficult, and he felt his outward reaction of pain was unacceptable for a male, and that it had made him weak in Christina's eyes.

He realised that the meetings with Joan were probably at an end, but despite this he waited the next day at the same spot hoping she would be there. Sadly, he realised that she would never come again and resigned himself to that. It was a bitter blow to him, having had such optimistic aspirations about the so-called friendship that had been flowering between Joan and him. Its beauty had decayed in a short period of time and it was impossible to pick up the pieces, especially as he had been made to look so inferior.

During his school lunch break he would make a journey to the town centre. On his way there he would encounter Hannah walking in the opposite direction and initially attempted to acknowledge her as he passed. She avoided looking at him and eventually he accepted that she did not wish to communicate with him. Their paths invariably crossed like this every day, and these encounters were daily reminders of the termination of his relationship with Joan.

Chapter Three – Diversions

As the sea and all its associated attractions were in close proximity to the village in which Norman lived, it provided a welcome distraction for him from the familiarity of village life. He had explored the seashore on his own, after his mother had agreed to it. She felt he was capable of being trusted not to indulge in anything foolhardy at that age – his early teens. The shore after the tide had ebbed was particularly fascinating for him, and he derived a great amount of pleasure from investigating what creatures lay beneath the rocks which had been exposed by the outgoing tide. Beneath were crabs, starfish, anemones, eels, tiny fish and many other sea creatures. Particularly of interest were hermit crabs. Their ingenuity at acquiring such a comfortable home and the alacrity with which they withdrew into it when disturbed impressed him. It was comforting to observe how well protected they were, and they reminded him of his own insecurity in contrast to them. There was a beach about one hundred yards long, and a small pier was situated at one end of it. The rocks in the areas on either side of the beach had huge quantities of winkles attached to them. It felt to him that his frequent forays to gather them was contributing to the food resources of the home, and the fact that he was the only one in the family to partake of the winkles was a trifle disappointing to him.

His family depended on the area round about for survival. Each household had a croft in which the owners grew potatoes and corn. They also possessed a cow and some hens which provided milk, butter and eggs. A shop was available for the purchase of other groceries and basic items. It was situated half a mile away from Norman's home. The potato patch was quite extensive, and from it the family could be self-sufficient in that product for the whole year. The production of an adequate quantity of potatoes was carefully planned by each household. Enough potatoes were planted to provide a year's supply for eating purposes in addition to storing a supply over winter to plant the following year.

Norman experienced the potato planting for the first time when he was ten. It was facilitated by a tractor pulling the plough, creating furrows into which the potato pieces were placed. The procedure attracted a huge flock of seagulls, some of which alighted nearby.

'Why are the seagulls so interested in our efforts?' Norman asked his grandmother.

'They find it a struggle to survive, and are interested in anything which they would regard as food that might be exposed by the ploughing process,' she answered. She seemed to detect his apprehension of the unpleasant squawking that the birds produced. 'They communicate with one another in a way that differs from human beings,' she continued. 'They can still be successful in finding food for themselves.' She then quoted the Scriptures: 'Are not two swallows sold for a penny?'

This extract from the Gospels needed explanation, so she supplied the meaning to him. He had already read the Bible from cover to cover during a period in which he had been deprived of reading material, but found it difficult to understand. His grandmother reassured him that he would be able to understand it better after consolidating his English reading. At present he was to read material that he could cope with. It seemed a sad misfortune that in order to plant the potatoes it was necessary to destroy the carpet of daisies which proliferated over the area. 'To A Mountain Daisy', by Robert Burns, seemed to fit the occasion, although the sentiments of the poem could be applied more to a thousand than to one individual flower:

> Wee, modest crimson-tipped flow'r,
> Thou's met me in an evil hour,
> For I maun crush amang the stoure
> Thy slender stem:
> To spare thee now is past my pow'r,
> Thou bonnie gem.

The awareness of the fleeting nature of our existence is usually very far from the mind of a child, and the survival of the flowering plants in nearby fields consoled him. No thought of death disturbed his mind and he revelled in the present. Every day he would discover something even more wonderful than the previous day. Each day was enjoyed to the full.

Death was soon to affect Norman's life, through the demise of his grandmother whom he was very attached to. Very soon she started developing headaches, which were extremely severe. Eventually she became partially paralysed down one side of her body, was diagnosed as having suffered a stroke, and admitted to hospital. On the return of his mother from the town hospital where she visited her, he demanded his comics but was upbraided for not considering the plight of his grandmother, who was at death's door. The seriousness of the situation became apparent to him.

'Your grandmother is dying and you only have thoughts of receiving your comics! You should have shown compassion and inquired after her. She has a lovely caring nature, and in her pain and suffering had the presence of mind to ask after you.'

'You usually buy me comics when you visit the town,' he replied querulously.

'Not on this occasion. I had more important things on my mind. She will eventually be discharged home from hospital and I expect you to show her that you care for her when that comes to pass.'

Her tearfulness and distraught reaction made him realise that the stroke was life-threatening and he tried to subdue the feeling of disappointment he had displayed and replace it with something more appropriate to the situation. It had not been revealed to him that her illness was so grave and an attempt had been made to protect him from undue sadness.

'I am very unhappy that she seems to be so ill; I wasn't aware of the seriousness of the situation,' he replied.

That remark seemed to pacify his mother. She had the responsibility of tending to her own mother's needs, and a heavy weight lay on her shoulders at this time.

Eventually his grandmother was discharged from hospital to

her home. She was confined to bed and was administered sedatives regularly, but the prognosis wasn't very good. On one occasion when Norman was present at her bedside, his grand-mother said, 'Kiss my head, Norman.'

He obliged by stooping down and kissing her as she lay feebly with her head on the pillow. He was surprised at her fragility but felt confident that she would eventually recover. The prospect of her imminent death never entered his head. He found it difficult to show a lot of emotion as the situation was unusual for him.

'It's nice to see you back, Gran,' he said uncomfortably.

'Promise me you will be a good and obedient boy after I'm gone,' she said.

'I promise,' he replied, choking back his emotions, and puzzled as to where exactly she intended to go.

Soon afterwards her condition worsened again. He overheard his mother discuss her situation with a neighbour. 'The doctor regrets to say that she has only a matter of hours to live. I cannot bear the thought of her leaving this world but am consoled by the fact that she will experience a new life with Jesus in heaven. Our life here hardly begins when it is finally demanded of us.'

> I trace the rainbow through the rain,
> And feel the promise is not in vain,
> That morn shall tearless be...

Her companion could have quoted this before adding softly in a hushed tone, 'Her pain has lessened considerably since the administration of the sedatives.'

'I pray that her suffering will come to an end. Her breathing is shallow and laboured and that signifies how close to death she is. She is the dearest person in the world to me. I shall miss her dreadfully,' his mother replied.

Norman was forbidden to survey his grandmother as she lay dying in another room, as the experience might be too traumatic for him, so eventually he was sent to bed, where he lay awake for several hours, churning over in his mind the fight for life that was happening in the adjoining room. It seemed as if she was reluctant to loosen her fragile hold of life and clung precariously to it, as evidenced by her efforts to breathe efficiently. She seemed to be making a superhuman attempt to maintain her breathing, shallow as it was. However, within a short time she went from this world and into the next, despite all efforts to extend her life for as long as possible.

'Swift to its course, ebbs out life's little day…'

'We won't wake him to tell of her death, but will update him tomorrow morning after he wakes up,' his mother said, addressing her companion who was present with her in Norman's bedroom.

Norman wept silently with his face hidden underneath the bedclothes and tears poured down in floods, wetting the flimsy sheet which covered his head. He was left to come to terms with his grievous loss on his own, preferring not to reveal his emotions to the couple who were briefly present in his room. He felt an emptiness that seemed could never be dispelled, as there was no one who could replace his grandmother in his affections. Her love for him had been patient and kind, and she had shown the depths of her love in many caring ways. She hadn't been able to lavish much on him in the material sense, as they were below the poverty line, but she made up for it in the giving of herself. Her presence in his life could not be replaced.

Eventually, after a restless night he was wakened by his mother, who gently informed him of the death that had occurred the previous night. She tried to break it gently to him, but was unaware that he knew of his grandmother's death about the time it happened. There was no comfort available that could lessen the blow. He felt the world would never be the same again.

'I have arranged for you to have breakfast with a neighbour before you make your journey to school, as I have to plan for your grandmother's funeral,' she said. 'I hope you have learnt something about relationships from your experience of my mother's love and kindness to you. She was the most important person in the world to me, and life will never be the same again to me. Try to pick up the pieces of your shattered life.'

'This is a completely new experience for me,' he replied. 'I have never before been robbed of someone so close to me by death.'

The neighbour welcomed Norman into her house and added some words of comfort as she prepared his breakfast. He sat benumbed, oblivious to her crumbs of comfort, while she set out breakfast before him. He surveyed the plate, on which lay two softly cooked fried eggs and some boiled cabbage. Unfortunately he hated softly cooked eggs and his hatred also extended to boiled cabbage. He made a feeble attempt to take a mouthful but found it an impossible task. He eventually had to make the excuse that he was so affected by the recent death that he felt unable to eat. She swallowed this excuse after an initial reaction of annoyance.

It took many years before the memory of his grandmother faded from his mind, but time is a healer. People in that kind of situation have to continue with their lives, and though initially there is sadness and despondency, the deceased person is replaced by others in their thoughts and lives.

A neighbour called Kenneth was instrumental in introducing Norman to the sport of fishing. The interest he took in fishing was helpful in replacing the sadness at the recent bereavement in his family by something he found exhilarating and relaxing. Kenneth had a spare fishing rod that he offered Norman, who accompanied him to an area of cliffs about a mile's walk away. Kenneth promised Norman that he would make this a regular occurrence every Saturday; during the week he was self-employed as a fisherman and had a part share with his two brothers in a fishing boat. When they reached the summit of the particular cliff that had been selected, they had to make their way down to the base of the cliff. The height of the cliff was about a hundred feet and the way to the base mainly consisted of a grassy area. However, towards the end of the descent they had to negotiate a rocky area, Kenneth leading the way. Norman experienced a feeling of trepidation during this part of the descent, mixed with keen anticipation of the fishing that lay ahead.

'Always concentrate on your descent, using your hands and feet to aid you, and don't be distracted by anything,' Kenneth said. 'There has been a case of a villager who went fishing to these parts several years ago and was never seen again. His body was never recovered.'

'It is easy to be distracted, as the seagulls are squawking and swooping so much,' Norman replied. 'There is enough evidence of their obvious proximity from their droppings, which have defaced the cliffs.'

As he spoke a seagull dived at them and at the last moment swerved away.

'It obviously has a chick nearby that it is protective about,' Kenneth explained. 'Let's make our way down as quickly as possible and evade its attention.'

The rock Kenneth had chosen was quite a popular fishing spot with the villagers and there were several hopefuls clustered together, leaving just about sufficient room for two more. The time had to be chosen carefully, as for some inexplicable reason the fish never fed on the ebb tide. Kenneth had chosen his time well as the tide was just turning to flow. There was no wind, and the sound of the waves breaking against the rocks was at a minimum. The rhythmic sound was extremely restful and soothing, and the wide expanse of sea all around served to add to the beauty of the place. There were some oily patches round the fishing area, the rest of the sea only slightly disturbed. Many years later Norman was reminded of the beauty of that environment when he heard his first live musical concert that included *La Mer* by Debussy. The following extract from *Kubla Khan* seemed relevant to Norman:

> Could I revive within me,
> Her symphony and song
> To such a deep delight 'twould win me,
> That with music loud and long,
> I would build that dome in air,
> That sunny dome! Those caves of ice!

Kenneth advised me on how to bait the hook, using a small amount of bait to attract a relatively small type of fish called pollack, whereas he used a larger bait and different tactics to lure the larger pollack.

'Your fishing rod is not strong enough to cope with landing a lythe (a large Pollack),' he said, adding, 'it would break. Leave that with me and concentrate on catching smaller fry.'

'No one has caught anything so far,' Norman replied. 'I might be the first. I am sure our fishing trip will be successful. Even if I fail in my efforts I will still have these beautiful surroundings imprinted for ever in my mind. I find this activity so relaxing.'

'Make sure you maintain the bait at a sufficiently long distance from the seaweed that is extending from the rock,' Kenneth advised. 'You do not want to get it snagged there, for then you would lose your tackle.'

The trip actually ended with success for Norman, who managed to catch six pollack, whereas Kenneth left empty-handed. The catch was sufficient to provide a meal for all the family, being gratefully received as they were struggling to make ends meet, and the fish were greatly appreciated as a result. Norman felt a sense of achievement at his efforts. Kenneth almost became like a father substitute to him, as he would often spend Saturday evening conversing with Norman's mother. Norman somehow felt that Kenneth's rapport with his mother was instrumental in forming a close bond between Norman and himself.

True to his word, Kenneth faithfully took Norman fishing every Saturday, and each time introduced him to a different rock, some that were quite difficult to scale. The direction of the wind made some more suitable than others, and even in extreme conditions there were always some rocks that were fairly sheltered from the wind. A turbulent sea in the proximity of the rock made it impossible to catch anything. As time went on Norman lost interest in fishing for small fry and his quarry became lythe, which are large pollack about the size of a small salmon. He started going on his own for that purpose during the week, and ventured far and wide to do so. He had to make the most of it, as the fishing season was from June to October.

He felt increasingly isolated from his companions because he had started feeling there was something different about him which set him apart from others. His interest in fishing served to isolate him even more, and although he enjoyed it, it was a lonely pursuit. It replaced his football activities with his associates, which occurred every evening after school. Children and young adults were literally obsessed with football in those parts, being little different from anywhere else. The countryside afforded the choice of several football playing areas, of which they had several favourite pitches there. Norman and his companions congregated together and chose two teams which competed with one another until one side reached a total of twenty goals. The pitches were small, so it wasn't impossible to achieve that number of goals inside several hours. Norman tried to be superior by playing with the outside of his right foot, but unfortunately he began to be less and less valued as a good player as time went on. Eventually, when teams were selected he was almost the last to be chosen. He had always regarded himself as a good player but now the sad realisation dawned on him that he was no longer any good at the game.

This failure at football, the experience (real or imagined) of his school friends' reaction to his rheumatic chorea, and his recent awareness of the fact that he was illegitimate, all combined to make him feel desperately unhappy at times. His feelings seemed to be justified on one occasion when walking down the pavement during the school lunch break. He noticed a nurse approaching him who had been partly responsible for his care during his stay at hospital for the treatment of his chorea. At the same time he was aware of children walking some distance behind him, laughing among themselves. He sensed that they might be poking fun at him but did not want to betray any visible feeling of distress, as the approaching nurse might think he was displaying weakness. She kindly stopped to talk to him and eventually departed. He felt comforted by her attention, but the behaviour of the boys made him feel doubtful about his interpretation of other people's actions. At school there were a few pupils who came from the same village as himself, and he never found out whether they had divulged to the rest that he was illegitimate. He felt certain they had revealed it and felt betrayed; whether the suspicion was justified or not, he never found out.

Meanwhile his new found interest in fishing blossomed and flourished. He had forsaken his delusion of being a skilled football player and devoted his leisure time to the sport of fishing. Even when indoors he busied himself making flies, and if the weather permitted he would go to his usual haunts, fishing again. His only problem was being certain of a regular supply of fresh mackerel for bait; this was not guaranteed, as the fishmonger's van sometimes sold herring only. When mackerel wasn't available he had to resort to other lures like flies or artificial rubber eels. They weren't as effective as mackerel. He was guaranteed his favourite bait on Saturdays, as Kenneth invariably brought some back home after his week's fishing in his boat, and accompanied him rock fishing on that particular day.

One Saturday, on a particularly stormy day, there was only one rock suitably sheltered from the wind, so they decided to go there. They had been there on a previous occasion when Kenneth had caught seven lythe ranging in weight from six to twelve pounds, and it was tempting to try and repeat that success. The only problem was that the rock face was crumbling and it had to be negotiated with care. They were unsuccessful on that occasion as far as catching anything substantial, having to be satisfied with a dozen small pollack. They had hardly just started to ascend when Norman heard a shout behind him, and on looking back he realised that Kenneth had fallen a distance of about fifteen feet onto a rocky ledge. It later transpired that as he was endeavouring to pull himself up on his ascent the rock that he was holding crumbled and gave way, with the result that he fell that distance.

'Can you get up?' Norman asked. 'Do you need any help?'

'I think my eyesight has been affected,' Kenneth replied. He went on, 'Let's make our way to the top and leave the fishing rods and catch behind. I want to make sure I have two available hands on the way up.'

'I can carry both rods,' Norman suggested, but Kenneth insisted on his initial command.

'We'll make our way to the nearest house and you continue down to the telephone kiosk and phone for an emergency doctor, while I remain in the house.'

Norman ran the half-mile to the nearest kiosk and, never having used a telephone before, he had to summon the shop-keeper next to the kiosk to make the call. The shopkeeper criticised Norman for being unable to use the phone, and that was the beginning of Norman's fear of using a phone, which would surface in later life during his future employment. Norman had attempted to make the call himself but had been unsuccessful.

The call was eventually made and a doctor summoned to the house where Kenneth had remained. The first outcome was that Kenneth had not suffered any serious injuries, and was allowed to go home under his own steam. The second outcome was that he vowed never to go rock fishing again, and he kept his word. On the Monday following, Norman returned to collect the fishing rods, which had been abandoned on the rock face. He was surprised to observe that the catch had been eaten by seagulls despite having been attached to the rods with a piece of string; the fish heads were left still attached.

The danger that was associated with rock fishing affected Norman personally on one trip. Kenneth, no longer feeling inclined to accompany him fishing on Saturdays, was only involved to the extent of recommending such-and-such a rock to visit, after taking the weather and tide position into consideration. On one such Saturday Norman found himself fishing on a reef, to which Kenneth had suggested Norman go and to which he had given directions to find; Norman had never gone there before. He spent several unfruitful hours fishing, and the tide had risen by about ten feet during his stay there. He resolved to give up his attempts to catch anything and made his way along the reef to what he hoped would be dry land. Unfortunately, the rising tide had separated the reef completely from the land and there was a long, ten-foot-deep stretch of water barring his way! He had never swum in his life, but had the presence of mind to undress and make a bundle of his clothes. He then managed to float across the gap by clinging to kelp that was attached to the sea floor and floating upwards from it in a vertical position. He used it to make progress towards land which he finally reached. His clothes had become completely wet and after wringing them he dressed and made his way home, his wellington boots squelching as he went.

As Norman preferred to go fishing rather than associate with his companions, he felt a feeling of isolation that was accentuated by what had occurred on that day. The fact that he had had a near encounter with death magnified it, as he had been acutely concerned about his own survival. If he had drowned it would have meant an end to his feelings of inferiority. His aspiration of becoming a skilled fisherman seemed doomed to failure as well.

In the distant future he would have hopes to become a fisher of men through setting a good example as a Christian. A catch of one would have been acceptable. However, he had to confront Kenneth and his mother with nothing for his efforts and so invented a lie to suggest some amount of success. He claimed he had caught two lythe which he had attached to his rod to facilitate his 'swim' to dry land. He added that unfortunately they had become disconnected during his efforts to reach land and had floated away. He wanted to build an image of himself as an efficient fisherman to replace his shattered dreams of being a skilled football player.

His estrangement from his previous boyhood companions seemed to intensify as he became increasingly preoccupied with his diversion of fishing. The situation seemed to become more immediate to him when he encountered them one evening on his journey back home from fishing. They were enjoying a game of football, but Norman made a detour past them, keeping at a distance from them. One of them shouted to him in a humorous way, 'Have you caught anything?'

'I have only caught one small fish,' he replied, trying not to betray his embarrassment in the tone of his voice.

He felt a loneliness and separation from his previous associates that was hard to bear. He had made his decision. His separation from the others seemed complete at this point of time. His relationship with them had reached a new low, and the sad fact was that he was acutely aware of this and attributed it all to discrimination by others based on his being illegitimate. The probable reality was that any strained relationships between him and the rest of the youths was due to his faulty personality and oversensitivity. His poor catch on that occasion made him feel even more inferior. The chorea he had developed several years before was still haunting him, and he was convinced that that made a negative impact on his relationships due to real or fancied reactions from all those around him.

The sad fact that his family were about the poorest in the village added fuel to the fire, as far as it appeared to him. He was extremely aware of his family's poverty, their lack of adequate toilet facilities, and the dilapidated state of his home, which badly needed repairs to the roof. Sometimes he felt a strong feeling of despair when it rained – which happened quite frequently in that part of the country – and when the numerous leaks in the roof became apparent. However, life could sometimes be happy for him, as well as sad, and he felt some degree of security due to his mother's care and attention to all his needs. The absence of a father need not have proved insurmountable, as his mother supplied as much care as two parents. His state of mind was due to his extreme sensitivity.

In his late teenage years his grandfather suddenly developed a stroke. That was brought home to Norman when his grandfather was on his knees during the nightly prayers. It was the custom in their home to have evening prayers led by his grandfather. On this occasion, however, his grandfather remained speechless and unresponsive in a kneeling position, with the Bible opened in front of him. He was unable to continue his prayers, and eventually Norman's mother assisted her father to bed.

'You mustn't mock him – he is seriously ill,' she explained.

'He made us stay in a kneeling position for half an hour!' complained Norman, who had always felt a strong dislike coupled with contempt for the old man ever since he had struck Norman several years before.

'He needs medical treatment as a matter of urgency,' she replied firmly, and added, 'I will phone for a doctor tomorrow.'

The usual doctor had his practice seven miles away, and she was reluctant to summon him at that late time of night, preferring to wait till the morning, when he would be more disposed to make the journey. Although Norman had had a bad relationship with his grandfather, he still felt a twinge of sympathy for him that night.

That Norman was no longer given the opportunity to release bitterness and hate on someone had now materialised, as his grandfather had become completely paralysed, bedridden, and unable to communicate. Looking on his helplessness as he lay immobile in bed one could only feel pity for him. The care required for his continued welfare had become the responsibility of Norman's mother, who carried out her duties to him stoically as his daughter. To prevent bedsores from appearing on his body she had to turn him periodically in his bed without any help. Norman could have volunteered to assist her, but he felt a lingering distaste for his grandfather that prevented him from aiding her.

In later years he would look back on the circumstances with remorse, feeling that he could have been more helpful in the situation that had come about. On one occasion when an older friend and he were present in the room where the invalid was lying motionless in bed, the older companion remarked, 'Look into his eyes, and ask him whose son you are.'

'I can get no response,' Norman replied, having carried out his friend's instructions, and having gazed at the blueness of his grandfather's eyes, which seemed somehow to express disapproval to him. Remorse and pity flowed into Norman's soul, and from that time he regretted the past bitterness that had hindered a positive relationship in the past with his grandfather. There was no hope of a recovery, according to his mother; he would eventually die; his life had ended as it began as a baby; he was now completely dependent on others for his continuing life; his own state was simply reduced to automatic breathing, and nothing was voluntary.

> Swift to its course, ebbs out life's little day,
> Earth's joys grow dim, its glories pass away.
> Change and decay in all around I see,
> Help of the helpless, O abide with me.

The years rolled on, nearly four actually, until his grandfather died. Throughout that period his daughter had faithfully cared for him with compassion, sometimes addressing him as 'her little baby'. He had been the only male adult in the home, but Norman had rejected him right up to the point of his death. It was fortunate for his dependants that the cost of his funeral was covered by an insurance policy. The funeral took place in a graveyard five miles distant, to which the mourners were conveyed to by bus, and Norman had been requested to accompany them, which he did. The graveyard was overgrown with profusely growing grass that reached waist height in places. Obviously it was believed there that once death had claimed a person, it was unnecessary to tend the grave, as from that point onwards the deceased person would be in heaven or in hell, and nothing could alter that. What really mattered was living a Christian life on earth and committing that life to Jesus. The deceased person in question had clearly been in that category during his lifetime.

The grave had already been dug and the coffin was lowered into it. The process of lowering it seemed to accentuate the feeling of Norman's alienation from the deceased, and when the coffin had lowered completely, it seemed to him impossible now to make amends for his life of conflict with his grandfather.

'Pick up some dust from the ground and throw it on top of the coffin.'

A voice intruded on his thoughts. On obeying the person's instructions, Norman was hoping that this action would hide his pleasure at his grandfather's demise from those surrounding the grave. It had been a difficult struggle for him to appear suitably sad and bereaved at the death. He felt acutely that he was being a hypocrite and was concerned about whether his emotions could be sensed by those around him. Later concerns in the future about whether people could sense his true feelings when he was attempting to hide them might have originated about that time. His hands were soiled with dust and he was unable to wipe them clean. This seemed to take on a special significance to him as it seemed to draw attention to his apparently unsuccessful attempt to put on a show of sadness. However, once the funeral was over he was able to exclude all thoughts of his grandfather from his mind and continue with his life as if the old man had never existed.

Chapter Four – Immersion in School Life

Norman's success at his studies was limited. Mathematics was his special joy, and he would spend hours attempting to solve mathematical problems that appeared in his school books. Finding a proof gave him a feeling of satisfaction and pleasure. He excelled at this subject, the sciences being his favourite subjects. His vocabulary at this time was very limited and skill at languages was lacking as well. However Latin was an exception as he found its logical framework appealing to him.

Although he was poor at English he found literature and poetry rather interesting. The Shakespearian play that his class studied for their examinations was *Hamlet*. Hamlet's character fascinated him and his teacher discussed Hamlet's personality as he saw it, in great detail, over a period of nine months. Aware that despite his own shortcomings there was something special and dignified about the human person including himself, the extract that he found most relevant was Hamlet's utterance:

> What a piece of work is a man, how noble in reason, how infinite
> in faculties, in form and moving how express and admirable, in
> action how like an angel, in apprehension how like a god: the
> beauty of the world, the paragon of animals!

He would often look back at this quotation for comfort in situations where he experienced feelings of inferiority and lack of confidence. His future religious convictions would serve to support his views that human beings were set apart from other creatures and were made in God's image. There seemed to be something limitless about man's intelligence and capabilities that became even more apparent to him in later life, after his detailed study of Mathematics at university. Even the lowliest of persons demanded respect and he was always conscious of this fact. In fact the following extract from a hymn he took literally:

Let holy charity
Mine outward vesture be,
And lowliness become mine inner clothing;
True lowliness of heart,
Which takes the humbler part,
And o'er its own shortcomings weeps with loathing.

He could see that virtue in others but was uncertain as to whether he possessed it himself. He seldom looked analytically at himself, preferring that application to be addressed to his mathematical studies.

His period at school eventually ended and after the examination results were released he was accepted as a Mathematics student at Aberdeen University. There was a gap of three months until the University opened so he decided to find a temporary job until then. His first step was to sign on at the local employment exchange where temporary employment as a general worker in a hotel was offered to him. The employment officer mentioned that several of his school colleagues had found work as a group in another hotel prior to entering university. This made him feel excluded but there was compensation due to the interview that was arranged for him with the manageress of the hotel.

The interview for the vacancy he applied for went quite successfully. There was no thought in his mind that he might be rejected; he displayed his confidence by swinging his leg lazily too and fro, prompting the interviewer to admire the new pair of trousers he was wearing for the occasion. She decided to offer him the job at a salary of five pounds a week, an offer he was glad to accept. The conditions of employment meant that he would have to live in, with Saturdays free.

On his first day at work the manager of the hotel went over his responsibilities and did this quite thoroughly. Despite this some of his duties remained unclear to him. One of his tasks was to run out any excess oil accumulating in the boiler every morning. Unfortunately the quantity of oil that he extracted each morning was insufficient and some weeks afterwards the boiler stopped functioning. The hotel was thus deprived of hot water for a while until it was repaired later in the day. Only oblique references were made about his contribution to the boiler's breakdown and he got away lightly with it. The threat of dismissal hung over him like a cloud from the time of that incident onwards. One of his tasks was to polish the shoes of the residents who placed their shoes outside their door last thing at night. Unfortunately this was something he had never previously had experience of doing as his mother had taken responsibility for that at home. The amount of polish he applied to the shoes was excessive and he was unaware of the fact that it had to be rubbed until none of it was visible. Again there was no serious complaint, so he felt he was just about tolerated there.

Another of his duties was to carry the bottles of alcoholic drinks from the cellar to the bar after they had been selected as required for the day by the manager. After the basket had been filled it was customary for everyone concerned to sit at a table and relax with a drink. The manager's two sons would help him and on one occasion one of them became abusive, excessively using the word 'bastard'. Norman was never offered a drink at these meetings and after hearing the abusive words that he felt might be levelled at him he could never again relax in their company. In any case the son guilty of this behaviour seemed partially drunk. The incident served to create a permanent chasm between him and the others.

One morning, on leaving his hotel room in the morning to shave in the bathroom before starting his work, he was surprised to find Mary, one of the female members of staff lying on the stairs with her bust partly exposed. After unsuccessfully exhorting her to arise he became more and more aware of her state of undress and his hand hovered over her bust but never actually touching her skin. A voice from the top of the stairs interrupted his thoughts and said 'She's drunk. We'll see to her.'

'Why is she lying there?' he asked, not understanding how she had been able to remain in such an apparently uncomfortable position overnight as the voice had suggested.

'We will help her up the stairs,' they said, adding, 'we'll make as little noise as possible in case the manager hears us and discovers that she is drunk.'

Later on that morning it was revealed to him that the

manageress had discovered that the girl had come back drunk to work and had reprimanded the girl for this behaviour. He wondered if she had noticed how beguiling she had appeared to him in that position on the stairs. Later on in life he would come to the conclusion that the incident had been contrived to test his reaction with the opposite sex. It was difficult to erase the attraction he had felt from his mind and his relation with her became very strained, up to the point of his departure from the job. Every time their paths crossed he would become suffused with desire for her as he would automatically recollect her exposed breasts in her position on the stairs. However, although he basically found females physically attractive, he was always conscious of some imperfection in their appearance that disappointed him. No one was perfect to him; he felt he was aiming too high as far as the appreciation of the female physical appearance was concerned; they all seemed imperfect creatures to him.

Eventually his time there came to an end. He had continued to work up to a week before he was due to leave for university. As he was leaving the hotel for the last time he met Mary outside.

'Why don't you remain with us?' she asked.

'I intend to depart to start my studies at Aberdeen University,' he replied, adding, while trying hard not to reveal his distaste at this suggestion, 'My job here was only a temporary one.'

'Why are you going there? You have a good job here. How will going to university benefit you?'

He was amazed at her apparent ignorance of life and replied that going there and acquiring a degree through studying would equip him to be in a better position to find a well-paying occupation later on in life. He found the very thought of remaining in the hotel extremely distasteful but was diplomatic enough not to reveal this either by word or expression. Eventually they departed and he never saw her again.

Eventually the day dawned when he would have to leave his home to explore life at Aberdeen University. His one large suitcase was lovingly packed by his mother and she gave him some essential advice about how to cope in the world that awaited him. Afterwards he was to look back at these moments and wish that she had stressed to avoid leading 'the primrose path of dalliance' in later life. She should have mentioned the 'dangers, toils and snares' that awaited the naïve and inexperienced in later life but she probably did not want to discuss matters on which she felt embarrassed about due to her own experiences. She gave him a peck on the cheek; even that restrained show of affection seemed excessive to him; he was unfamiliar with even that degree of physical affection but would always look back at that parting with happiness due to his mother's display of love. The last thing he did before leaving the house was to kiss goodbye to his two pet cats. He was sadly aware that they were destined to be put down, as the home was to be abandoned and the other inhabitants were due to move permanently to London.

It was the custom there for people who were leaving the island for other distant parts to say a quick goodbye to all their neighbours. He was delighted about the realisation he made that some money was often offered to the departing person by the neighbours concerned. He decided to make an extra addition to the number of visits to say goodbye to a married lady whose beautiful blonde tresses had captivated his heart and mind. He had admired her from a respectable distance in the past and wanted to see her for the last time. When he entered he realised that her husband was present. They left it to him to generate some conversation but this was beyond him. 'I am feeling rather tired, Norman, and want to retire to bed. You'll have to excuse me. My daughter Chris is out.'

Her teenage daughter was a very attractive blonde, and Norman could hardly have failed to notice this. She was just eleven and had beautiful long plaits down her back. He had tried to suppress any admiration of her appearance in case his feelings would be misconstrued. Her mother's comments had put him in an awkward position. There was an uncomfortable period of silence which he eventually broke.

'I have to go now – I am sorry if I have disturbed your peace and quiet.'

It had become transparently obvious to him that there was to be no welcome or monetary gifts offered here, so he took his leave. He decided not to pay a visit to his best friend's home – if he could be called a friend. Norman lacked the commitment to establish a proper friendship with him as he regarded him with derision due to some character weaknesses on the part of his 'friend'. However, the 'friend' Donald was caring enough on his part to accompany Norman on the bus and say goodbye to Norman at the harbour from which the ferry was to take him to the mainland, on a journey that would last several hours.

Before this event Norman's last farewell visit was to a cousin called Marianne. She was an unmarried mother with two children, and Norman had always found it awkward to relate to them despite his blood ties with them. He tried not to show his feeling of disdain for them which he felt about himself as well. Marianne's daughter Mary was present with a neighbouring friend called Christine.

'Have you ever kissed a girl before? Now is your chance,' Marianne said, with the awareness of what teenagers consider as being of paramount importance in their lives. She offered her daughter's lips to him, but Norman was completely ignorant about what a kiss of that sort should involve and his efforts were feeble to say the least. It was not a pleasant experience as he had looked down on her in the past due to the fact that she was illegitimate. He had despised himself first, before anyone else in the same position. His simplicity about sexual matters was incredible at that time. He obtained more enjoyment from planting a kiss on Christine's cheek than kissing Mary. Unfortunately the first real kiss he would experience in life would be with a rather immoral woman, who for some inexplicable reason reacted positively to him on saying goodbye to him.

At the point where the ferry docked Norman said his good-byes to Donald and to Norman's sister Ann who had come there to say goodbye. He boarded the ferry carrying his excessively heavy suitcase down into the interior of the vessel. He vainly tried to find a lounge or somewhere to deposit his case but was completely unable to find his way around. Eventually he decided to make his way to the upper deck of the ship where he was exposed to the wind and the waves breaking over the side of the ferry. He remained there for the six hours the ferry took to make the journey, and until the day thankfully dawned – the vessel having left on the previous night. During the night a girl who had been on the same class as him at school emerged on to the deck and began to attempt to relieve herself there. She suddenly noticed Norman looking at her and exploded into a torrent of abuse using freely the word applied to people who were illegitmate. It was a journey that haunted him for the rest of his life.

Chapter Five – University

The ferry docked after a traumatic night weathering the storms on deck, and the train into the mainland was waiting to be boarded. Norman chose a compartment in which two of his schoolmates were travelling; they were also destined for Aberdeen to start their university careers there. Norman confided in them that he wasn't sure how he would know when the train would reach its destination, but they assured him that Aberdeen would be the last stop. Sure enough, the train finally drew up at Aberdeen station and Norman hailed a taxi that took him to his lodgings; he had arranged to stay there where bed and full board was supplied, having been sent with a list of suitable places to stay by the university in the summer. The reason he had selected this particular accommodation was that the cost was just within his range. He was relying on a grant of £80 a term from the Scottish Education Authority, which would be handed to him in the form of a cheque from the authority when he had matriculated. He was naively over generous with his tip to the taxi driver, giving him what amounted to double the fare. This was because he was so relieved he had made his way successfully to his destination, having never travelled in a taxi before.

On ringing the door bell, an elderly lady opened the door and greeted him warmly and invited him in.

'My name is Florence,' she said, 'and I hope you had a pleasant journey.'

'I had never been on a train or ferry before, so the journey was a bit arduous for me,' he retorted, not wishing to dwell on his unpleasant experiences, in case it would reveal his simplicity.

'This is John – he will be your room-mate. He is a fellow student who has decided to study French. There will be a third student staying here whose name is James, and I will be expecting him to arrive tomorrow. He is to be a student of history. Come in and I will make you a cup of Bovril. You can unpack later when you have recovered from your trip.'

Norman felt it difficult to relate to John, as his course was in the arts. He longed to meet his fellow students of mathematics. The university was due to open the following Monday, and he had arrived early on Saturday. There were no ferry trips from Lewis on Sundays as the islanders were intensely religious, a feature of their religion that forbade them from doing only that which was absolutely necessary on Sundays. After he had consumed his cup of Bovril he felt refreshed, and John was asked to take him and show him around the immediate locality, including the site of the university, which was five minutes' walk away.

As they were walking along the pavement he was very much aware of the busy streets that made such a complete contrast to the streets of Stornoway, which boasted only two sets of traffic lights in the whole town.

'What arrangements are made for washing clothes here?' Norman inquired. 'Will the landlady, Florence, be prepared to do this?'

'No. There is a laundrette nearby in which you can do that. Their charge is quite reasonable.'

The thought of exposing his dirty clothes in public deterred Norman from making use of the laundrette. In addition to that, he had never used one before, and was nervous about investigating on his own, as John did not take him inside. John probably assumed that Norman was not unfamiliar with laundrettes. Crossing the road and avoiding being run down by the traffic became a major problem for him for many years; he lacked guidance from anyone; how to cross a pedestrian crossing was beyond him.

That night he found to his distaste that he had to share the same bed with John, as there was only one double bed available in the bedroom. During the night he positioned himself on the opposite side of the bed from John, as far from him as possible. Norman stayed facing away from him all night. It was an unpleasant experience and was a situation which would arise in later years in different lodgings. Apparently Florence wanted to make maximum use of her facilities and create maximum income for herself through letting her rooms out to boarders. The situation seemed quite innocent to Norman and, although he found it unpleasant, no thought of impropriety was aroused in his mind. Apparently some students were packed together like sardines and were taken advantage of by enterprising landladies.

Next day, James, the third boarder, arrived. He discussed his course with Norman and showed Norman James Joyce's *Portrait of the Artist as a Young Man*, the study of which was part of his course. He asked Norman if he would be interested in reading it and Norman agreed. Joyce's relationship with the prostitute Rosie O'Grady made a permanent impression on his mind, and he was to regret afterwards not discussing the outcome of such a relationship with his room-mates. That the writer was prepared to reveal his clandestine relationship to the public surprised Norman at the time, as he felt he would have tried to hide it if the same experience had happened to him. Those who discussed the incident of sweet Rosie O'Grady with Norman seemed more knowledgeable about sexual matters than him, and he felt a trifle inferior at not having first hand experience in these matters. He felt that they suspected that he was still a virgin and tried to give the impression to them of having dabbled in those affairs in the past. The fact that he was able to make a relevant comment on the book gave him some encouragement. The discussion turned to the name Stephen Daedalus, which was attributed to the person telling the story, and Norman revealed that where he came from everyone had a nickname.

'Would you have used an assumed name if you had written the book?' John asked.

'No,' Norman retorted, and continued, 'I never liked my own nickname, nor would I want to hide behind another name.'

Norman had led a more or less morally blameless life up to that point, but had he foreseen that future events in his life would make Joyce white as snow in comparison to him, he might have hesitated in his reply.

'Let's give Florence's husband a nickname,' said James. 'Let's call him Geo.'

'Why call him that?' asked Norman.

The dictionary was consulted and it transpired that 'geo' was a word denoting a blowhole. It seemed that as weathering took many years to form a blowhole, so 'Geo' had developed into what he was over a very long period of time as well. 'Geo' and Florence were both retired pensioners who were trying to augment the income from their pensions by taking in some students as lodgers.

Some weeks after the university opened for students, John and two friends of his suggested to Norman that they should all visit an establishment that provided drink and dancing. They all sat at a table and each bought himself a whisky. William, one of John's friends, suggested that each of the four should contribute half a crown to make up a sum which was placed at the centre of the table. The motive for this seemed unclear to Norman, but he went along with the suggestion not anticipating that he was to wave goodbye to his own half crown. Four matches were removed from a matchbox and one was broken in half. William drew the short match and claimed his prize – a harlot who was hovering over the table asking us to buy her a drink. William scooped the four half-crowns into his possession and made off with her, having the courtesy to invite her to dance with him before the transaction was finalised. At that, Norman objected and requested his money back, but was told in no uncertain terms by the others that they had assumed he knew what was intended. It was many years later that the penny clicked for him.

Norman, not having had much access to the cinema before starting university, decided to make up for lost time. Instead of attending his practical classes in physics and geology he preferred to spend that time in visiting the numerous cinemas in that city, in the afternoons. His studies were neglected and eventually he received a letter from the Physics Department asking him to attend the next practical class as a matter of urgency. This he did, and the lecturer spoke to him as follows: 'Why haven't you appeared at the practical class in the last six weeks? You are only allowed to miss six classes at most. If you miss any more you will be failed in your subject and will have to leave university. Do you understand? What is your excuse?'

'I enjoy visiting the cinema. I did not realise that it was an essential part of the course to attend a certain amount of practical classes. I assumed that attending the lectures was sufficient.'

Norman made an effort to attend regularly, but one factor made it very difficult for him. He was unaware of the position of the nearest toilet to the practical class and was often unable to control his need to urinate. Excessive embarrassment about these matters made it difficult for him to inquire about their location, and so it was not unusual to see a pool of urine in the class when he was present. On one occasion when he was entering the main door of the building that housed the practical class he noticed a pool of fluid in the entrance. A female fellow student asked him if he was responsible and he denied it. She was good-humoured about it and addressed him affectionately. Her attitude helped to make him more at ease in that particular class.

Smoking twenty cigarettes a day amounted to one of the few vices he had. To him, smoking seemed to be a desirable and essential pleasure and he felt it placed him at the very least on a par with his fellow students. He would proudly light up his cigarette after leaving the lecture hall but one day he lit his cigarette in the lecture room after the lecture had finished. On replacing the spent match in the match box so as not to litter the floor the hot match ignited the rest and the box burst out into flames. Thankfully, no one noticed this fiasco, as the lecture hall had emptied and the lecturer was absorbed in dismantling some remaining objects relating to the experiment he had been conducting.

His management of his grant was very unwise due to the excessive amount of money thrown away on cigarette smoking and the cinema. He was, however, very much aware that it was vital to pay his landlady her rent regularly each week, and this he did without fail. He depended on her to provide him with his meals – apart from the midday meal which he had in the University Union. He felt he owed her more than what the rent covered, and the feeling of being indebted to her made him feel uncomfortable. James and John were close friends with one another and he felt a trifle excluded. The evening meal in the accommodation that had been provided was not as a rule very appetising. On one occasion the meal consisted of a mixture of mashed potato and mince, the mince being restricted to an isolated lump here and there, making an insignificant contribution to the mashed potatoes. Norman delicately toyed with his food and came under the scrutiny of Florence.

'I have noticed that you do not seem to be enjoying your meal,' she said, adding, 'if you do not like it you can leave it. Do not feel you are being pressurised to eat it.'

'I am sorry, but I feel full up,' Norman replied lamely.

She did not propose to provide him with any other food to replace that which he had rejected so he had to remain hungry throughout the rest of the evening. He had been surprised at how effortlessly his two fellow lodgers had consumed their meal, and this made him feel even more excluded than ever. Florence's disapproval was apparent in her cool attitude to him that evening. At least Norman displayed some gratitude for his nightly cup of Bovril and this – at least in his mind – seemed to pacify Florence.

When the end of the term came, Norman was impelled to seek refuge with his mother and sister, who shared an attic room in his aunt's house in London. He was unable to exist financially in Aberdeen as he had nearly spent his grant by the end of the term, after which were four weeks of Christmas holidays. This aunt, who was named Chrissie, was married to an Irishman named Pat, and they lived in a large house whose rooms they let out to lodgers. Pat made an attempt to find Norman temporary work during his stay in London, by accompanying him and visiting neighbouring factories, and asking if they had any vacancies. During one such unsuccessful morning Pat took Norman for a beer in a nearby pub.

'You seem to me to be unconcerned about the future,' Pat said. 'What will happen if you do not succeed in finding work for yourself during this vacation? I hear that you do not have the money available at the moment to cover the cost of your fare back to Aberdeen. You can stay with us free of charge in the meantime.'

'I am confident things will turn out for the best eventually,' Norman replied, adding, 'I've never tasted beer before. It tastes delicious with this cheese roll.'

The conversation turned to women and Pat asked tentatively if Norman ever had relations with a girl.

'Have you met any nice girls at university? There must be plenty suitable girls there for you...'

'No,' replied Norman, 'girls are very few there. The vast majority of the students are boys, but there is one girl that I like enormously who is positioned next to me at the weekly chemistry practical. Her name is Gillian, but I have never been able to summon up the courage to speak to her.'

The conversation ebbed and flowed for half an hour, after which they returned home.

Next day a telephone call was received from his mother's relative, Bella, inviting Norman and his mother to visit them. They made the journey that evening and were welcomed by Bella and led into the house. Rosie, Bella's daughter, whom he regarded as nice acquaintance, welcomed him warmly. She showed a deep love and affection for him that he found very unusual for a member of the opposite sex. He was overcome by her enthusiasm and warmth.

'How do you find being a student at university?' she asked him. 'What subjects are you studying? I hope you will be a success there.'

'I am studying mathematics,' he replied. He went on, 'During my first year I will be studying other subjects – physics, chemistry and geology – to broaden my knowledge of science. I always enjoyed mathematics at school, so I decided to study the subject I liked best. I did consider becoming a doctor but was ignorant of how to proceed with applying for studying the discipline of medicine.'

'It was lovely to meet you,' she said. 'Do you like Coke? I will go out locally and buy a bottle for each of us.'

Norman offered to pay his own share, but Rosie insisted on buying the drinks out of her own pocket. She returned, and they continued their conversation sitting opposite each together and relishing their Cokes at the same time. It was intimated to him by his sister several years afterwards that Rosie and he had the same father. At that particular time he was unaware who his real father was, as his mother never discussed the matter with him. It was a subject he found too embarrassing to broach with his mother, so he remained for many years ignorant of the fact. He was overwhelmed by Rose's friendliness and found himself admiring her appearance and especially her voice, which was soft and slow. She was the most beautiful female he had ever seen and he admired her enormously. He tried to hide his feelings for her in her presence as he felt she would disapprove.

Bella's male friend, Bill, decided to make an entrance at that point. Bella's husband – and Norman's father, it transpired later – had been admitted to a mental asylum, and she had befriended Bill in her husband's absence. He revealed that he had arranged for an interview between Norman and one of his previous employers with a view to hiring Norman as a temporary street cleaner.

'Don't mention to the person who interviews you that you are a student and that you only want work for a month,' Bill said.

'Thank you very much,' Norman answered. 'This stroke of good fortune has appeared in the nick of time as I am down to my last penny. I hardly have sufficient money left to pay for my fares on the buses here.'

'I will provide you with the directions of how to get there. The interview is scheduled for tomorrow morning at 10 a.m. Be sure you arrive on time. The result is a foregone conclusion, as I have used my influence to guarantee you get the job.'

Next day Norman appeared as requested for the interview and was given the job, starting immediately. He was coupled with an obese man named Tom who dragged behind him a barrow in which the rubbish was to be deposited. Norman was supplied with a brush and swept the pavements, depositing the leaves and other rubbish in the barrow as he went along. At one point he came across some dog faeces on the pavement and asked Tom whether to leave them there or whether to add them to the rubbish accumulated in the barrow so far. Tom said that it was necessary to remove the mess from the pavement as well as all the other debris that had been discarded there. It seemed a trifle degrading to Norman, but as the job was only temporary and job satisfaction was immaterial he felt he could tolerate it for a month. Tom seemed to relish in his role as instructor and left Norman to do all the sweeping.

A few hours later it was time to call in at a local café for a cup of tea. Tom had a pack of sandwiches with him but Norman had come unprepared with nothing. Norman ordered his cup of tea, producing a silver Scottish threepenny piece to pay for it. He was taken by surprise at the reaction of the cashier, who told him in no uncertain terms that that particular Scottish coin was unacceptable in England.

'You have a cheek thinking you can sneak a foreign coin to pay for your cup of tea! You will have to supply me with acceptable tender. I have made your tea. That will be threepence please – in the right coinage!'

'I am sorry,' Norman retorted, 'I have no more money in my pocket. You will have to provide that cup of tea to someone else.'

'Anyone else want a cup of tea?' the cashier asked.

Norman sat down with Tom, who bought his own cup of tea and proceeded to devour his sandwiches. After a few minutes a cup of tea was placed in front of Norman, courtesy of a sympathetic customer who had witnessed the dispute. Norman thanked the customer profusely and pondered why his tea had been provided by a stranger rather than by his workmate, Tom. The incident drove a wedge between him and Tom which Norman found difficult to tolerate. Relations between them deteriorated from that time onwards.

Eventually Norman's period of employment neared an end. Shortly before this happened the weather worsened, and within a short time that area of London acquired a covering of snow and the pavements iced over. It was impossible to clean the pavements under those conditions, so Tom and Norman had to resort to scattering sand and grit on the pavements to help pedestrians to negotiate them. On one day the couple were joined by several more men and, equipped with pickaxes, they strove to clear the pavements of ice outside an underground station. Norman's efforts to wield his pickaxe were practically futile, as he found he couldn't apply enough strength to make an impact on the icy pavement. He resorted to observing his companions in their work, leaning on his pick axe as he did so. Unfortunately the foreman happened to arrive at that time and exhorted them all to 'put their backs into it'. Norman was glad when the time came for him to complete his temporary job. He had been successful in saving enough money for his fare back to university for the second term of study.

When he returned to his lodgings in Aberdeen he happened to mention to his room-mate in a superior sort of way that he had gainfully passed his vacation in employment. When the type of employment Norman had been occupied with eventually transpired, his room-mate asked sarcastically, 'Did you have to clean the dog faeces from the pavements?'

'Yes,' Norman retorted, adding, 'I had to accept the job because there was nothing else available.'

'I would never stoop to such a degrading job! Weren't you capable of finding anything more dignified?' he continued.

'I had to accept it; otherwise I wouldn't have been able to return to university, as I had no money for the fare.'

His room-mate could see the logic of that statement so he ceased to voice his distaste for that type of work.

Norman had accompanied his aunt's husband, Pat, several times to greyhound racing in London. The actual races were very exciting to him and a casual bet of a shilling now and then added a bit of enjoyment to these occasions. He happened to see grey-hound racing advertised in one of the local papers in Aberdeen, so he decided to pay the stadium a visit one evening after his daily studies at university. He decided to place a bet of two shillings on two dogs, but for some unexplained reason the cashier advised him to change his bet to another pair of dogs. Norman complied, and it was with a sense of profound joy that he came back to the cashier for his winnings of £3. She seemed to be as delighted as he was, and congratulated him on following her instructions.

When he returned to his lodgings the landlady asked how he had fared in his visit to the greyhound stadium. Norman was exuberant about his success, and when he confided to Florence how much he had won she suggested to John that he accompany Norman there next time. This suggestion was rejected vehemently by John, who stated that he would never stoop to that sort of recreation. It seemed a disparaging remark to Norman, who was well and truly put in his place. This reaction made Norman feel that he was somehow regarded as an outsider there and it served to make him more aware of his shortcomings; it drove a wedge between him and the other occupants of the house; the comment made him more isolated there.

It was a difficult exercise for him to commit all his studies to memory, and as a result his performance at geology and chemistry was poor, whereas the subjects of physics and mathematics, which involved to a large extent logical thinking, were more of a success for him. The cinema occupied a lot of his time, and he did not devote enough time to his studies. He was pleasantly surprised at his performance in physics for the class exam, the results of which were displayed on the notice board at the beginning of the second term. Although his marks were below 50% his actual position was midway down the list as many of the other students had low marks. He sensed that the Physics tutor was pleased with his results, as the tutor selected him on one occasion to explain, in front of the class, the reasoning behind his solution of a problem set as homework. It concerned the solution of a problem relating to the motion of an ice skater.

'The centre of gravity remains constant due to the fact that friction is negligible,' Norman blurted out.

'Can you enlarge on that?' was the reply.

'No,' Norman tersely retorted, feeling utterly terrified at the prospect of prolonging his address to the class.

'Thank you. Your evaluation of the problem was accurate. You may return to your seat.'

Norman crept to his seat feeling sick with embarrassment. He was relieved that the ordeal was over and attributed the amused reaction of the class to the fact that he was illegitimate. He even felt that illegitimacy could exclude a person from university and felt that in his case this rule had been inadvertently overlooked. Later in life he would look back with disbelief at his approach to life at that time, as when he reached middle age these inferior thoughts would largely disappear.

When time came for Norman to leave his lodgings the land-lady had a dispute with him regarding the rent. He felt he shouldn't have to pay for the coming weekend, as his departure was on a Friday. She insisted that he pay the full week's rent, so he eventually complied. At the door when he departed she intimated that he would not be welcome back the following year.

'Is it because I am illegitimate? I feel others deride me because of that.'

'No, Norman, it is nothing to do with that.'

She provided a blanket for him to cover his body on his journey down south.

'You do not have to return it,' she added.

He made his way down to London to his stepfather's flat, his mother having married a civil servant with whom she had been corresponding when she had lived up in Scotland. She was relieved that due to her marriage she would be moving into more comfortable accommodation. This was understandable, as her home in Lewis had been virtually falling down over her head, and she probably felt that she and her husband would become closely attached in time. Their flat was a huge improvement on the attic room in which she had previously stayed with her sister. Harry, his stepfather, along with his mother, greeted him warmly at the door. After entering he was ushered into the living room and a box of cigarettes indicated to him.

'I made sure that they are your favourite brand,' Harry said, adding, 'help yourself to them while we prepare a meal for you.'

'Thank you very much. I appreciate your generosity.'

Norman had arranged an interview with a security organisation with the intention of paying for his expenses in London during the four months' summer vacation. He had arrived in London penniless. Fortunately for him the interview was a success, and he was employed as a temporary security guard in a factory some distance from his accommodation. It would never occur to him that there might be a possibility of not finding any work, as he regarded London as a place of many opportunities. He felt no doubts about the future, feeling confident that the future would be bright as long as he was successful at remaining at university.

On his first day at work, his work associate showed him the areas of the factory he should patrol. They had to wait until the all the factory workers had left before they could do this. Each point had to be registered on a paper roll with a numbered key. After a couple of attempts Norman was left on his own to conduct the patrol. Apparently he had remembered most of the points, as his associate remarked at a later date that the paper roll had been examined and most points had been registered.

Norman had bought an end-of-year university magazine and proudly spent his time reading it during his free time at the factory. It was a humorous magazine, and although the majority of the jokes were beyond his appreciation he still uttered a forced laugh after each one he completed reading.

'This is a funny one. What do you call a clown carrying a nun on his back?'

'I don't know.'

'Vergin' on the ridiculous.'

Norman's grasp of English was so poor that he was unable to associate 'virgin' with 'vergin' '.

On the days Norman had free from work, and he had three free days a week, he maintained his interest in the cinema. He had read in a newspaper a year previously about the legalisation of prostitution in London and this had attracted his interest. As he was still a virgin he desperately wanted to have a relationship with the opposite sex, but did not know where and how to approach a prostitute. He had read that the West End and Cable Street were riddled with prostitutes and so several times he scoured these areas in the dark hoping to find one. He was terrified of being noticed, especially by a policeman. His attempts to find a female to have sex with failed. The words of the hymn, 'I heard the voice of Jesus say, "I am this dark world's light",' should have been heeded by him. Those areas made their own substantial contribution to the dark world in which he lived.

His mother's relationship with Harry had struck stormy waters before they were married. Afterwards she revealed that during their engagement he was so devastated at his mother's death that he exclaimed that he was going to commit suicide and locked the door of the bathroom after entering it to carry out his threat. His mother tried to conduct a dialogue with him from outside the bathroom and when this proved futile she struck the glass door with her fist in desperation. Her hand was badly gashed and at that point Harry exited from the bathroom and voiced his concern for her injury. It was necessary to visit hospital to have it treated. Norman always felt that that incident showed his mother in a good light.

Norman succeeded in finding alternative accommodation for his second year at university. He shared a room with another second year student called John. Relationships with John progressed in a satisfactory way – or so it appeared to Norman – until Norman happened to make a remark to him addressing him as 'John'. John rounded on him in fury and said viciously, 'Don't call me by my Christian name again!'

Norman felt devastated at this retort and there was no further conversation between them. The incident had destroyed their relationship as room-mates. Mealtimes in the lodgings were a very tense affair. The landlady obviously found it hard to make ends meet as the meals provided for her two lodgers were meagre. Her husband sat at the end of the table enjoying an appetising meal while they, on one occasion, were provided with grated raw carrots on toast. At the end of the first term Norman was asked to leave, but the landlady provided him with the address of a family that were prepared to take him in as a lodger.

His new landlord belonged to a strict Christian sect and the other lodgers were all working class. He was kind enough to take Norman as company on a fishing trip to Kintore with expectations of catching trout or salmon. Norman was allowed to take over several times and the landlord was kind enough to instruct him regarding baiting the hook and general technique. As a result of this fishing trip, Norman resolved to buy a rod from a fishing tackle shop, soon after they returned to his lodgings. He asked for advice from the shop assistant and settled for the cheapest rod in the store. He was assured that it was suitable both for salmon fishing and trout fishing.

He ventured on his own to Kintore several times and once caught six trout. He offered them to his landlady and they were specially cooked for next day's supper. He felt as if he had accomplished a lot, and the occasion reminded him of the piping in of the haggis on Burn's night. Those gathered round the table received their trout, but Norman was disappointed that the meal consisted of a single fish on a plate allocated to each person without any accompaniment of vegetables or potatoes. It was no surprise in a way, since the meals there were usually as basic as those consumed by Van Gogh's 'Potato Eaters'.

He managed to make a relationship with Leslie, one of the lodgers. Leslie had obtained information that Norman was inexperienced with the opposite sex and decided to solve this by taking Norman to a pub frequented by prostitutes. They sat down and discussed women in general. Leslie informing him that sometimes women were in the habit of approaching tables seeking 'customers'. After a long wait, prolonging their drinks for as long as possible, they decided to leave.

'It is better that you should meet a girl whom you can fall in love with and enjoy a good relationship with. Not everyone can enjoy making love to a prostitute. You are better of not consorting with them.'

'If I came across one I would yield to temptation,' replied Norman, who felt disappointed at not encountering one. He felt no antipathy towards prostitutes at that particular time in his life, and would have echoed the words of Jesus: 'Let him who is without sin cast the first stone'. Prostitution and adultery were of the same gravity to him; they were both forbidden and regarded as sin by the vast majority of people.

He reached his 21st birthday during his stay at the lodgings he had been sent to. As he was a long distance from relations he assumed the day would pass like any other day for him. It happened to come to the landlord's attention that that particular day was his 21st birthday and, observing a letter on display in the lounge, Norman asked if it was an intended birthday card for him. The crestfallen look on his face when it proved not to be his betrayed his feelings. As a consolation the landlord asked two young female residents to celebrate his birthday over a glass of Coke. They all sat round a table, but the females were tactless in their conversation and one shook the bottle of Coke and released the contents, which spurted out.

'Is this something you do every morning?' asked one.

Norman responded by bursting into tears. He felt completely humiliated. It was impossible for him to find words to reply to this accusation and he fled the room. His birthday celebration had been a disaster. He had felt superior to the working class people he shared his accommodation with, as he felt he was privileged in being a university student. He was wildly wrong in his attitude.

This experience dented his feeling of superiority and drew attention to what he regarded as a misdemeanour on his part. A sense of humility was what he lacked. The following biblical quotation from Mathew seems to be apt at this point: 'Therefore, whoever humbles himself like this child is the greatest in the kingdom of heaven.'

That winter, through his Christmas vacation, was severe. The snow lay on the ground in great drifts. He had succeeded in finding temporary work as a relief postman and struggled through the inclement weather for a month delivering letters. Christmas arrived, and the lodgers were asked to make their own arrangements for that day, as the landlady wanted the day for herself and her family. On Christmas Eve Norman had done his customary delivery but had been unable to complete his delivery of all the letters. Some were remaining and he resolved to deliver them on Christmas Day. Dutifully he went out to fulfil this resolution, tramping through the snow and slush in his efforts to deliver the remaining letters. The snow permeated through his shoes and he could hear the joyful noise of festivities from within the houses. In the end he had to abandon his delivery and the following day he discarded the remaining letters in the refuse bin. The shops were all closed and he was unable to buy any food for himself that day. The day had turned out to be a nightmare for him when it should have been a joyous occasion.

He got into the habit of buying an occasional bottle of lemonade which he used to consume at night. On one night he drank excessively and during the night he experienced what seemed like enuresis, thoroughly wetting the underlying sheets. He decided to remain quiet about it but was confronted by the landlady about the matter after she had made the beds in the early morning. He was unprepared for her reaction; she told him to leave immediately. However, she had arranged for him to reside at a private hotel where they were willing to provide him with lodgings. His new landlady asked him on arrival why he had left his previous accommodation. His reply was that he had been drinking the night before and had subsequently been 'sick on the bed'. She seemed to accept this explanation and welcomed him into his new abode.

He completed his course, after three years, being successful in completing his ordinary degree. He sailed through the final exams but needed a slightly higher mark to continue to do an honours degree, so he decided to retake one of them in September before the new session in October.

He kept in touch with his mother but was not a very regular communicator with her. He was surprised one day to receive a letter from her saying that he lacked concern, as she had to have a Caesarean operation to enable her to give birth to her son, Iain. She claimed that she had almost not survived the ordeal. Norman had been completely kept in the dark about her pregnancy. He suspected that it might have occurred to her that Norman might have been jealous if he had been told. No other plausible explanation came to his mind. Looking back at this time Norman would realise that he had had been so involved in his university career that he had made little communication with his mother. No wonder she wrote as she did.

'I hadn't been aware that she was pregnant. The father isn't really mine,' he confessed to his room-mate, Jim, suggesting vaguely that he might be illegitimate, and feeling interested in how Jim would react to this comment.

'It must be difficult for you to have received that news out of the blue,' remarked Jim, not revealing any sense of superiority in his reply.

At the completion of his third year he made his way to London again, where he could be close to his relatives, including his baby half-brother. He managed to find accommodation in the form of a bedsitter, the landlady of which was Polish and very attractive. Her husband, if she had one, was absent from the house; the only other presence was that of her son.

Chapter Six – Subsequent Developments

He was fortunate in being accepted by the security firm he had worked in the previous summer, and was able to exist on the wages he received from them. He was based in a well-known high-rise building, working with about five others, patrolling the place during the night. One member of the group would prepare an appetising meal later in the night, and this was approved of by the security firm, and was free of charge. There were about a dozen cleaners who worked through the night in their employment there. One of them was on friendly terms with Norman, but he felt superior to her due to her lowly occupation. How wrong he was in his attitude to his fellow human beings! One of his fellow workers, James, was on particularly good relations with a black cleaner, who also appeared very attractive to Norman. On one occasion they were both in the same lift as Norman travelling up to the top floor, which was about the twentieth. During the lift's progress, Norman happened to look round and noticed that the black cleaner was partly exposed and that James appeared to be making love to her.

'Keep your eyes on the floor indicator. We don't want to miss our floor,' James said.

Norman obeyed without making any comment on the incident he had witnessed. He was shocked at their behaviour, finding it very distasteful.

On his penultimate day working for the security firm, Norman felt sleepy and exhausted. It was approaching daylight and he decided to abandon his position at the desk temporarily and catch up on some sleep. Only a short time had elapsed when he was awakened by James and told to go back to his post. He was soon summoned to the security superior, who bluntly told him that he was sacked. Apparently James had divulged Norman's absence from his post to his superior. The security firm were decent enough to drive him back to his bedsitter personally.

'Have you just one shift of uniform?' the man asked Norman as he drove him back.

'Yes,' replied Norman abruptly, feeling annoyance at himself and at the man driving him home.

'You were entitled to another. You can keep the trousers,' the man replied.

The situation caused Norman such depression that he really felt life was not worth living. He would have ended his own life if it could be accomplished painlessly. Ophelia's descent into madness would soon overcome him as well, though he had not the courage to terminate his own existence. No elaborate ending for him, he thought; just do it without leaving any details of the motive.

> There is a willow grows aslant the brook
> That shows his hoar leaves in the glassy stream;
> Therewith fantastic garlands did she make,
> Of cornflowers, nettles, daisies, and long purples...

He had sat his exam again, successfully, and was given permission to continue his studies towards an honours degree. He returned to the same hotel to which he had been recommended by his previous landlady. The food there was reasonable and a lounge was provided for the guests, and a television included. A lot of his time in the evening was spent watching it and his studies took second place. Despite his addiction to television he succeeded in coming first in the class in functional analysis and received a first class certificate for that year.

One of his room-mates was a music teacher who got him interested in classical music. Norman enjoyed the music provided so much that he purchased a record player. Lawrence, the music teacher, was so enthusiastic about music that some of his enthusiasm rubbed off on Norman. Another student sharing his room was called Peter. Peter noticed that Norman enjoyed reading books on chess, so he suggested they join the University Chess Club. A competition was organised between the student members and Norman progressed to the semi-final, when a foolish sacrifice of his knight for two pawns cost him the game.

He was very disappointed and could never accept a defeat at chess without feeling that his defeat was due to the fact that his logic had been badly flawed.

On another occasion a girl student in thigh boots turned up at the chess club and created a buzz there. Her dress was very provocative and Norman could scarcely stop himself from casting lingering looks at her. To his disappointment she never even looked his way, although he desperately attempted to make eye contact with her from a distance.

He managed to find new lodgings again when the end of his fourth year at university dawned. It was a squalid place barely fit to be described as lodgings. He shared the room with a student who had attended Edinburgh University and was lodging there until the next term started. Norman felt a common bond between them because of that. Norman's acquaintance related to him how he had replied to an advertisement for accommodation. He had been surprised, when he phoned the number supplied, to hear over the telephone a female voice, who professed she was a prostitute's maid and described the prostitute – with some amount of exaggeration as it turned out. Norman was asked if he was interested in the phone number. Norman needed no cajoling, so he professed his interest in visiting this prostitute and was handed her telephone number.

Norman went next day to a telephone kiosk and duly dialled the number he had been given.

'The lady is twenty-one and is very attractive, and the basic rate is two pounds,' a voice at the other end said.

'What is her address?' Norman asked without exploring the situation any further by asking for further information.

He made his way there and rang the bell of a basement flat. The door was opened by a middle-aged woman who ushered him in. Norman mistook her for the prostitute and was eager to 'conduct business' with her, saying so using the minimum of words. He was ushered in, and shortly a woman in her forties made an entrance, only partly clothed.

'My name is Jean. The price is two pounds.'

Norman extracted two pound notes from his pocket and handed them grudgingly over to her.

'Most of my customers offer a tip to the maid. She depends on tips to augment her income.'

'Will half a crown be sufficient?' Norman asked.

'Yes,' Jean replied, adding when she had received the total amount, 'take your clothes off.'

'I have never had sex before,' Norman admitted.

The business arrangement was completed, but to his bitter disappointment something seemed incomplete and unsatisfactory about the experience. He had omitted the foreplay, as he was aware that Jean almost certainly found the proceedings and him repulsive. He received little satisfaction from it and left after politely saying goodbye. She said she hoped he would come again, but he felt it was strictly business with her. When he returned to his lodgings he went to the lounge, and strangely on *Top of the Pops* they were playing 'Satisfaction' by the Rolling Stones. He was told that the lounge was only for permanent residents and to leave the lounge. It seemed to him that his escapade was known even by the Rolling Stones, or at least by the occupants of the house he dwelt in. He felt like quoting to them the advice given to Ophelia by her brother Laertes, as Norman sensed they were quite possibly immoral themselves and hypocritical.

> Do not, as some ungracious pastors do,
> Show me the steep and thorny way to heaven,
> Whiles, like a puffed and reckless libertine,
> Himself the primrose path of dalliance treads...

He persevered in visiting Jean, hoping something positive would result from his association with her. He felt all that was needed was a personal relationship with her and that then the rest would follow. She did co-operate by engaging him in limited conversation after every visit, but he did not achieve any lasting enjoyment from the relationship. He felt like commenting to her, 'Then neither do I condemn you. Go now and leave your life of sin.' Norman hoped that Jean could be coaxed to abandon her life of sin as a prostitute. He hoped that one day she would come to her senses, hopefully like the kept woman becomes aware of her sinfulness, as depicted in 'The Awakening Conscience' by

William Holman Hunt. The woman in the painting renounces her immorality and makes a decision to leave her sinful life behind her.

Eventually he turned to someone new, and an advertisement in a shop window stating the sale of two kittens, one black and the other white, appealed to him. It was obviously aimed at those who were interested in consorting with prostitutes, as the whole of the window was devoted to similar suggestive advertisements. He made the necessary telephone call and arrived at the brothel hoping that his fortunes would change.

'What would you like?' asked the white kitten.

'I would like to express an interest in the black lady,' Norman replied nervously, anticipating an increase in the price.

'No problem. The price is two pounds.'

He felt relieved at the arrangement thus far, and the lady was ushered in. He did not receive any response from her either before, or during, or afterwards. It resembled a union with a statue of a Roman goddess – beautiful to look at, but having no feeling or responding pleasurably. He would have preferred it if there had been more females from whom to choose from – three at least. He could take on the role of Paris, who was depicted by Rubens in his painting 'The Judgement of Paris', and award the golden apple to the most beautiful of the goddesses he was judging. Although in the situation that presented itself to Norman he had nothing to give apart from the agreed price of the transaction, what he expected to get from them was not the rotten apple he received. The prostitutes were hardly Rubenesque, but appeared to him more desirable than the goddesses in the painting, as the latter were over fleshy.

'Would you be interested in pictures?' the white kitten asked, adding, 'You can take part. You have the necessary qualifications.'

'No thank you,' he replied. Even he felt shocked and repulsed by this suggestion. On his way out he noticed the black kitten glued to a television as if it was all in a day's work. She didn't even respond to him when he said goodbye. Not yet quite feeling deterred, he continued to visit various prostitutes, one after the other, until finally he decided to stop and resolve never to do it again. He had committed this sin only for a limited period of a few months, but would bitterly regret his past when becoming a Christian. He would be comforted by the fact that people who had more glaring sins could repent of them and lead a new and transformed existence.

He felt he was living a double life. His sexual entanglements were unknown to those people he knew in Aberdeen. He returned after the summer holidays to start the final year of his honours course in Mathematics. There was just one girl on his class. He happened to notice her one day walking in the quadrangle with a male friend. Norman felt the urge to stop and admire her from a distance but their eyes met. At that moment he was reminded of the prostitutes he had known, because of his fellow student's revealing dress and her white stockings. The thought came to him that his covert sexual life might possibly become apparent to people in general, but after weighing things up he thought it unlikely.

His studies were divided into seven units, and his favourite branch was functional analysis. He had not kept up with the work in algebra and was woefully behind in numerical analysis as well. Fortunately, he was able to answer some questions in the final examinations which were based on the previous year's studies. On the last day of the examinations, which consisted of a unit on numerical analysis – his worst subject – the supervisor had occasion to leave the room for a short time, trusting that the students would not cheat. Norman felt the impulse to clarify some vague point with the nearest student, who gave an ambiguous reply. The thought that this had become known to the supervisor haunted Norman for a long time in his later life. His question was superfluous, as it was near the end of the examination and no information received could have been put to good use. It was a stupid thing to do.

Before the summer holidays Norman had a discussion with the head of the department about his future. Norman said he would be interested in doing an MSc in functional analysis if he got an upper second – which was the minimum requirement. The head tried to dissuade him, suggesting instead an MSc in computer programming. Norman was not influenced by the head's suggestion, so it was decided to wait until the results of the examinations were known. A grant would then be applied for if necessary.

The summer vacation was spent in London. He had noticed an advertisement for a bed-sitting room on display in the window of the newsagent from which he had selected the phone numbers of prostitutes in the past. He vowed he would never visit one again. When inquiring about the vacancy he was met at the door by a middle-aged black man who offered him accommodation for a reasonable price. Norman had found employment during the vacation as an invoice clerk. This was sufficient to cover his housing costs, with not much left over for food and pleasure.

At the end of his first week in his new lodgings, he went down to Sam's room – he was the landlord and lived on the premises – and offered Sam his first week's rent. As Norman was on his way out, Sam suggested he come down later on and watch television with him. Norman needed no enticement to do this as he had been deprived of the opportunity of watching television for most of his life.

In the evening Norman descended the stairs and was admitted to the landlord's lounge, where he was offered a seat next to him in front of the television. The landlord intermittently engaged in conversation and the banter came round to a discussion of one's sexual inclinations.

'Are you a heterosexual?' Sam bluntly asked.

'I haven't really experimented properly, but I believe I am,' Norman responded.

'Women are unpleasant creatures,' said Sam. 'I knew a woman once who had to have an abortion. She agreed to this without considering the moral side of it. The aborted foetus was discarded like an unwanted physical object. That is what sex with women can lead to.'

He took hold of Norman's hand in his own and Norman instinctively withdrew his, feeling a sense of revulsion for the man. Sam suggested a glass of orange juice, to which Norman assented. Norman sipped the orange drink and soon felt a warm glow envelope him. At the time he didn't associate his feeling with the drink, but much later in life he looked back on the event and had suspicions that the drink might have been laced with an aphrodisiac of some sort. His resistance lessened. The following quotation from Gospels applied to him when he looked back on his sinful past; at least, that would be his hope. 'He who is forgiven most loves most.'

Soon after the start of his MSc course he was informed by the head of the department that he was not properly qualified to undertake it. This was because Norman had not attended the graduation ceremony in the summer, and according to the head he did not officially have a degree. He urged him to graduate in December, otherwise his MSc course would be terminated. Norman hadn't realised that attendance at the graduation ceremony was essential, thinking that his BSc would be conferred automatically on achieving the requisite pass mark in his exams. The possibility that he might have to abandon his mathematical career overcame him with terror, and that night he knelt on his knees before God and prayed fervently that he would be allowed to complete his course. It was the first time as an adult that he had prayed to God for help.

He had led a double life until this point, and the fear that somehow his sexual improprieties would somehow become revealed to his acquaintances at university invaded his mind. This fear was triggered by the head's remarks to him. The thoughts that all would be revealed crept into his mind, and people's behaviour to him seemed to confirm this. The difficulty he experienced in his role as a class tutor to first and second year mathematics students contributed to his mental decline. His most terrifying thoughts were that some student in the class would pose him a problem he couldn't solve satisfactorily. There was one group of students who were in the habit of laughing among themselves in one of the tutorials, and Norman took this personally and felt the laughter was directed at him, especially as one of the students had been one of his room-mates in the past. Norman thought the student would be more aware of Norman's background, having known him personally earlier in his career. The experience was frightening for him.

Norman received payment from the university for his work as a tutor. This was an important and vital addition to his grant, and he was able to afford the fee for hiring a gown for the graduation ceremony, which he attended in December. He decided to write a letter of denial of any wrongdoing and sealed it. He envisaged being exposed in public at the ceremony and was very apprehensive of the event.

Seated at the ceremony and waiting for his turn to be called, he decided to entrust the letter to a student sitting next to him, telling him to make the contents known if an example was made of him in front of all the other students. However, much to his relief the degree of BSc was conferred on him without any problem; when he got back to his seat he claimed his letter back unopened; he destroyed it later.

Chapter Seven – Descent into Schizophrenia

On his first meeting with his mother on his arrival in London for the winter vacation, he was so distressed and tortured mentally that he had to confide in her his fears that his private affairs had somehow been made public. As male relations between the same sexes were mostly illegal at that time, Norman feared that the police had been involved in a surveillance of him during the time that he had kept company with Sam. Norman had in fact been suspicious of the occasional flashes that occurred during these occasions he had spent with Sam, but had been reassured by Sam, who maintained that the television was faulty. Now Norman was of the opinion that pornography may have been suspected by the police and that as a result the lodgings had been bugged to ascertain for the benefit of the police what might have taken place. After his revelations, his mother immediately phoned for a taxi and accompanied him to Hackney Hospital.

On arrival at the hospital he was interviewed by a male psychiatrist, to whom he confided his suspicions about the police's real or fancied involvement in his affairs. Norman maintained that he wasn't a homosexual.

Another official made an appearance and advised Norman not to give any personal details to anyone else regarding his experiences. It was suggested to Norman that he remain in the hospital as a patient and that he would receive treatment there. Norman agreed.

Later on that day he was more exhaustively interviewed by a female psychiatrist called Dr Mica, whose Belgian accent he found irresistible. The conversation came round to sexual matters, when he voiced his concern that he might be regarded as a homosexual. She asked him if he had any grounds for possessing that point of view and after some hesitation he ventured to say, 'I once held... hands with some boys at school.'

'That wouldn't be interpreted as a homosexual act,' she said.

He sensed that she would become cold and distant to him if he was to be completely honest about his past, and that his attraction for her wouldn't be reciprocated. He remained as an inpatient and under observation during his vacation in London. No more discussions about his sexual life took place. He received occupational therapy while there, and on one occasion it was suggested to him that he play table tennis for recreation. He had never played before and it was decided that he play against a fellow patient about his own age. This person was quite familiar with the game and repeatedly returned the ball with such force that Norman was completely outclassed. He almost felt suicidal at his experience and eventually the occupational therapist replaced his opponent with a young female who was a beginner to the game as well. He enjoyed his game with her and felt the pleasure he had experienced had been reciprocated. Apart from his therapy and weekly sessions with Dr Mica he received no further treatment. There was no medication provided and his condition was tentatively described by Dr Mica as 'a persecution complex'. When the time came for him to resume his studies he made a decision to go back to the university for that purpose, with Dr Mica's approval.

On arriving back at the university he made contact with a mental health clinic that had been suggested by Dr Mica and waited in a room for the arrival of a psychiatrist. In the psychiatrist walked, mincing his steps as he came towards Norman, who felt convinced that his personal affairs had been revealed to the psychiatrist, who seemed to be mocking him. One of the questions the doctor asked was if Norman ever had felt sexually attracted to his sister. This was vehemently denied by Norman, who found the question deeply insulting. The interview was attended by a female psychiatrist as well, who seemed to have a permanent grin on her face; it seemed that she found Norman's sexual life something to be amused about.

The psychiatrist suggested a medication called stelazine and gave him a prescription for a month's supply. The medication had a soporific effect on Norman almost from the start and he found he could not tolerate the heavy leaden sensation in his head that resulted as a side effect. He decided to discontinue it and informed his psychiatrist of his decision.

Feelings of guilt about the past increased, and people's

apparent disapproval seemed to confirm his belief that his past sexual behaviour had somehow – possibly through his denials – become widely known by everyone in contact with him. Finding his suspicions hard to bear, he decided to test the waters by suggesting to the landlord that his son might be in possession of some personal information about him.

'What sort of information are you implying?' asked his landlord.

'That I have been guilty of misdemeanours in the past,' Norman replied.

'I am not aware of any such knowledge,' was the landlord's reply.

His inner torment became so acute that he decided that night to take an overdose of aspirin. He went to bed that night, not knowing if he would wake up in the morning. He felt a sense of relief when he eventually did wake up. However his overdose resulted in a ringing feeling in his head and ears that subsided as the day progressed. The landlady suggested he find new accommodation, as his ideas about her son were wrong. Soon he moved into the university's hall of residence – possibly being offered this accommodation through the efforts of his landlady to get him out of her home. The following biblical quotation from Luke's Gospel seemed to fit his past, when looking back on it as a Christian: 'Therefore, I tell you, her many sins have been forgiven; for she loved much. But he who has been forgiven little loves little.'

Norman's sins to him seemed huge, and the fact that he received forgiveness from God for them very much later in life seemed to put him in the category of loving much. At least he hoped so.

His depression and anxiety became so severe that he took a slight overdose of the stelazine as a cry for help. Again, there was no intention on his part to commit suicide. He got more than he bargained for, as the higher dosage of stelazine caused him to exhibit jerking movements of his limbs. The doctor was summoned and his psychiatrist arrived at the same time. Norman was confined to bed until the side effects of the drug diminished and he was capable of resuming his studies again.

His tutor, Dr White, had suggested a topic to him for his MSc thesis. It was suggested that he should combine some papers on interpolation with a recent paper by Lennart Carleson, who solved a problem in mathematics called the Corona Problem, and published a paper with his proof. Dr White had stated that Carleson's result might be generalised to functions on a group, and that this might be a suitable PhD topic. Norman had to admit that he had not applied himself to the study of algebra the previous year as he should have.

'I skived a bit in the algebra course,' he crudely confessed.

Dr White appeared shocked at this attitude and just suggested concentrating on the MSc only. He suggested to Norman that over the following three months he should read a book by Kenneth Hoffman called *Banach Spaces of Analytic Functions*. This book would be essential for Norman to understand Carleson's paper. Norman read a chapter a week and was told by his tutor to discuss any details he found difficult to understand. At the end of the first week he asked Dr White to clarify a point he had failed to understand. Dr White was of the opinion that Norman should have been able to understand the point and refused to help. Fortunately, Norman had only one more question to ask two months later regarding the contents of the book, and this question was answered in full by Dr White.

After the Easter vacation, it was time to tackle the papers on interpolation and the Corona Problem and combine them into a thesis. Norman's grasp of English at that time was poor, and he proceeded with his MSc by expanding all the unexplained details in the papers, enlarging them as much as possible. It was a very difficult task as the writers of the papers only supplied the basic essentials with little explanation. The papers on interpolation were straightforward. However, regarding the Corona Problem, Norman was unable to follow one part of the proof that appealed to the properties of Riemann surfaces, as he was unfamiliar with that topic and could find no clarification from other sources. This proved to be almost a permanent problem for him until he saw a way out a few years later when he finally submitted his thesis.

There were three other MSc students, two doing functional analysis and the other algebra. One of the former was a Chinese student called Stephen, who studied regularly with Norman in a room allocated for MSc students. His topic was one in which Norman was unfamiliar with.

At the beginning of the Easter vacation, the other three students went by train to London to attend a mathematical conference over a period of a week or so. Norman had not been invited by the head of the Mathematics Department, but Stephen had requested Norman to meet him at his arrival in King's Cross. Norman, Stephen and another friend of Stephen from the university – a Dr Chow – had a meal together in a Chinese restaurant. They conversed in Chinese for part of the time, which made Norman feel uncomfortable. After the meal was ended they offered to pay for it between them. Norman met up with Stephen on several occasions to show him round London. Stephen later admitted that he hadn't enjoyed the time much, but he did find a visit to a café near the House of Commons with Norman very enjoyable. They had a cup of tea and had a discussion on mathematics there.

At the beginning of October 1967, Norman completed his MSc course. Unfortunately the problem he had encountered in Carleson's paper prevented him from completing his thesis in time for the coming graduation ceremony, and so he abandoned it for the present, only to find a way around it when he had sufficient time to devote to it at a much later date.

His accommodation in London this time was in a hostel mainly for students. He had been allowed to return there, as he had confided in the manager of the hostel – a priest – that he had mental health problems and was without a place to stay. Full board was supplied but the food was awful. For a few days he shared a room with a black youth who was obviously mentally ill. The youth, on one occasion, confided in Norman that he had mislaid the five-pound note that he had set aside for his week's rent. Bidding Norman to assist him in looking through his drawers, the student flicked a five pound note, crumpled into a ball, in front of Norman. Without hesitating Norman placed his foot on the note and when an opportunity arose retrieved it from under his foot and retained it.

The next evening Norman broke into the note by buying

some sweets and was horrified to notice the black student and a companion emerge from the back of the shop. His conscience troubled him enormously afterwards. His behaviour seemed to him transparently obvious to all around him, like the clarity of Vermeer's 'Art of Painting', with Vermeer's precise use of light; only in this case the resulting effect was ugly. It was an incident that he never forgave himself for. It was fortunate for Norman that he could ask for forgiveness after he became a Christian, and that he would receive forgiveness before it was too late and suffer the following fate:

> The master of that servant will come on a day when he does not expect him and at an hour he is not aware of. He will cut him to pieces and assign him a place with the hypocrites, where there will be weeping and gnashing of teeth.

Norman had to find permanent employment and set about applying for a job, His first decision was to apply for a job as a lecturer in Mathematics, and so he sent in several application forms to various colleges who had current vacancies. His first interview after leaving university was with the Napier College of Science and Technology situated in Edinburgh. He received reimbursement for his fare so that he was not out of pocket by attending for the interview. He arrived in Edinburgh two hours before the interview and had a meal in a restaurant. The cost of the meal would also be reimbursed on production of the receipt. There were three applicants for two vacancies. When Norman's turn came to be interviewed he was ushered in to a table round which were seated the interviewers, one of which was the head of the college. The latter seemed to be rather dismissive and asked Norman how he would set about establishing a computer programming class for the students.

'I would learn it along with the other students,' Norman replied weakly, being completely in the dark about programming.

'Thank you for appearing,' the head replied suddenly, adding, 'you will be informed of the result in due course.'

After several more unsuccessful interviews with various colleges round the country, Norman decided he was not destined to be a lecturer and started applying for computer programming jobs. He was offered an interview with the Government Communication Headquarters in Cheltenham for a vacancy as a computer programmer. After being shown into the interviewing room, it transpired that the computer programming would be used to break Russian codes.

'That sounds exciting,' said Norman.

After the interview was over, one of the interviewers drove Norman back to Cheltenham station, asserting that many applicants were rejected if the references were unsuitable. He said that Norman would need a security check from MI5 and so it was arranged for an MI5, official to visit him at his mother's flat after the references were taken up.

Eventually the MI5 official came, and he seemed a jovial man.

'Is there any information on the application form that you would not want to be made public?' he asked.

'Yes,' said Norman, continuing, 'I would not want to reveal I am illegitimate.'

The man from MI5 was probably stunned by that answer. Quite possibly it had emerged during his prior investigations that Norman had a history of mental illness, and so would be deemed unreliable for a job like that. On top of that, he had asked if Norman had enjoyed his stay at one of the residences he had mentioned. This happened to be the one in which an attempt had been made to seduce him by his previous landlord, so he was possibly aware of that as well. He was invited to have a cup of tea and biscuits, an offer he eagerly accepted, demolishing several biscuits, and sipping his tea with his little finger elegantly curled round the handle of the cup.

Several weeks later Norman received a letter from Cheltenham turning him down and stating that there were no vacancies for him in the Royal Naval Scientific Service. This sounded like a broader exclusion than Norman expected, and he voiced his disappointment to one of the students in the hostel who had provided him with a reference.

Norman continued to work as an invoice clerk and made applications for professional work from week to week. His workmates commented several times on the fact that Norman had an honours degree in Mathematics but had failed to find an appropriate professional job. This put more pressure on Norman to seek professional employment, and this may have showed, as his previously solid relationships with them deteriorated into lukewarm ones. He could hardly wait to leave but had to remain in order to earn his living. It seemed to him that they sensed that he had just suffered from a mental disorder, and a serious one at that. The fact that he was aiming for a higher position drove a wedge between him and the others. The office manager had kindly offered to keep him on there if he felt that way inclined. He gave a polite refusal, as his established background of mathematics would have been wasted had he agreed.

One interview for a vacancy as computer programmer occurred with Standard Telephones and Cables. Norman was invited there for an interview. The initial interview was with the manager, followed by an interview and lunch with the senior programmer. Norman felt he showed innovation by choosing prawn balls as opposed to the pork chops chosen by another candidate who was present at the meal as well. Afterwards, the senior programmer confided in Norman that he would be chosen and led him back to a final interview with the office manager. However the manager's attitude was belligerent and he clearly disagreed with the senior programmer's decision, stating that he would not have Norman working on his premises, no matter what. His attitude almost precipitated a breakdown from Norman, who blurted out, 'Is it because I am illegitimate?'

He hoped that the reason for not being accepted was not his mental illness as he had made an indirect reference of it to the manager. The manager snapped back in no uncertain terms. 'I would not have you here on any account! You would end up sitting in a corner with the rest of your workmates shunning you.'

His words proved to be highly prophetic when Norman was eventually to find his first professional job. He was escorted out by the senior programmer and found it difficult to suppress his tears. It was the most disastrous interview he had so far, but he still felt it only proper to continue looking. The office manager had bluntly told him that he was incapable of doing a professional job and advised him not to make any further attempts towards that goal. Norman felt it to be inconceivable for him not to continue looking, so he maintained his attempts to find professional work.

After six months of applications and interviews he was finally offered a job as a computer programmer. He managed to get an interview with Elliott Brothers, whose naval division were developing computers for military purposes as well as manufacturing them in their own right. The assistant manager who interviewed him had asked him about his thesis 'Interpolations and the Corona Problem' and afterwards Norman felt that he had misunderstood the word 'interpolations', as this only referred to interpolating sequences not numerical interpolation. In any case, Norman had studied numerical analysis at university but had not applied himself to the subject. His appointment there was confirmed, and Norman said he would be able to start work in a week's time. The interviewer said that it would be necessary to sign the Official Secrets Act before joining.

The Friday before his first day at work in Frimley he arrived with a large suitcase in Aldershot, where he had decided to stay. He had been optimistic about his chances of finding accommodation but could only find temporary accommodation in a pub for a couple of days. Then he found a room in a small hotel in a small town near Aldershot itself. It had been recommended to him by the pub owner. The charges levied by the hotel were too excessive for him to stay there permanently, and so his stay there could only be temporary until he found a cheaper alternative.

Meanwhile he was encountering difficulties at work. On his first day he was introduced to his fellow computer programmers after signing the Official Secrets Act. A thick manual on machine code was produced and he was asked to study it and see if he could master it. When it came to be time for lunch he was invited to accompany the rest to a pub and have a snack there. They seemed to be friendly at first, but that came to an abrupt end. Next day he wasn't invited for lunch and was left on his own. The same applied every other day. Although he remained in that employment for a year he was completely ignored by the others, and was never again invited to the pub.

Trying to find a motive for their behaviour many years later, Norman feared that he might have expressed an admiration for

Hitler without realising that was contrary to the Official Secrets Act. It was true that at that time in his life Norman felt that Hitler had some good qualities, but later in life his views on the dictator changed and he realised that Hitler had been basically an evil man. His fellow workers' behaviour could not be explained otherwise, he thought. There was the possibility that his employers had unearthed the fact that he had suffered from a serious mental illness, and for that reason found him unreliable and not to be trusted. The manual he was attempting to understand was completely beyond him, and his employers decided to send him on a two-week course to their training centre in Borehamwood, with local hotel accommodation provided. The programming code quickly fell into place, and at the end of his two weeks' course Norman was quite familiar with it. When he arrived back at work he was asked to study a manual on Algol and this he did, mastering most of it. His first task was to change a program written in Algol to Machine code. After a day or two struggling with it, a girl arrived asking if he had completed it, but had to be told it wasn't ready. Next day he completed it and offered it to the manager. He thanked Norman and placed it in a waste-paper basket, or so it seemed to Norman on looking back.

An effort was made to find him a niche at Elliott's and he was approached by a programmer who went over some manuals on which he was working, that had to be approached using the tool of numerical analysis. Unfortunately it soon became apparent that Norman's knowledge of numerical analysis was inadequate and so that area of work was excluded to him as well.

Robert, the senior programmer, was Norman's immediate superior. He wanted Norman to help him develop a radar simulation program and filled him in on the basics. Various extras had to be developed into the program, so that it became more and more cumbersome and unwieldy. Eventually Norman decided to remain at work all night to complete the latest change, but when he presented the latest version to Robert, he was soon met by violent disapproval. Apparently it was rubbish – at least according to Robert. Robert had asked him to make a particular addition to it without supplying enough details on how to proceed. Norman had to refer to a book to get the information he wanted, but of course the best approach would have been a better dialogue between him and Robert.

Within a short space of time Norman's mental condition deteriorated. On a train journey to visit his aunt in London, he became acutely aware of a man reading a newspaper a few seats down the compartment. Somehow Norman felt that the man was inserting words into Norman's mind and instructing him to write them down. This Norman duly did and the end result was a poem of sorts, in which Norman had claimed to have killed his grandfather because the latter had terminated the life of Norman's ailing cat (this had occurred when Norman had been five years old).

At the present moment in time of writing the aforementioned facts, Norman realised that these events were practically impossible, for the simple reason that the man reading the newspaper had no previous knowledge that Norman carried a pen and paper on his person, so he could not have foreseen that Norman could have accomplished his instructions... Of course, if Norman had removed a pen and paper from his pocket to scribble on, the man could have had the opportunity to utter his instructions to Norman verbally. That would have been practically impossible as well, as the man was sitting several seats away and his words would have been overheard by others in the compartment.

One could go on analysing the incident indefinitely; there was a temptation to do this, as it seemed so real at the time. Of course there remained the unexplained reason why any man should behave like this. Why not reveal the information face to face? It was implausible now, but at the time Norman was convinced that his 'poem' had been revealed to him through this fellow passenger.

After arriving at the station he had a short journey to walk to his aunt's house. He felt a presence following him in the dark and felt that he was being followed. This made him focus attention on himself and he paused to examine the sole of his shoe. He found that the heel of his shoe had displayed a hole and immediately jumped to the conclusion that he had had a listening device attached to his shoe to reveal his whereabouts. He looked around him in terror but saw no one in the darkness. Eventually he arrived at his aunt's door – unannounced, and not having received an invitation to visit – and knocked. It was very late in the night and he had decided to come to his aunt because he felt that somehow she had the solution to his mental torment.

'Norman, what are you doing here at this late hour? Have you been ejected from your hotel?'

'I have been bugged! MI5 are tracking me to find out information about me. I have been assessed as a security risk where I work.'

'You are drunk, Norman. Come in and go straight to bed. You will be better in the morning.'

She ushered him in and led him to a spare bedroom, where he fell into a fitful sleep. He woke up in the morning and decided to allow his aunt to believe he had been drunk on the previous night. That was what she wanted to believe. He then quickly left and returned to his hotel in Aldershot.

Next Monday his mind was in turmoil. The fact that he was receiving very little assistance in his job as computer programmer made him suspect that his employers thought he was a security risk. He meditated on the 'poem' he had felt impelled to write in the train, and thought that might have some relevance to his present situation. He decided to confront his manager with the poem, and when allowed to see him he revealed to him the contents. It vaguely implied that Norman had been responsible for his grandfather's death. Norman could recollect his grandfather lying in bed with a stroke and unable to communicate. Norman could see himself in his mind's eye suffocating him with a pillow. The manager's reaction was one of amused disbelief, so Norman insisted on speaking to the person in charge of security. After Norman had handed the latter the poem, the recipient exploded in a furious outburst, asking Norman to get out. The manager insisted that Norman should be taken back to his hotel room in a taxi. The taxi was duly summoned and it made off in the direction of the hotel with Norman inside it. Norman, on some pretext, managed to get the taxi driver to stop, and then made his own way back to his hotel room, where he remained until an hour or so later. He then answered a knock to his door. Two men stood in the doorway.

'We are doctors sent by your manager at work and we would like to ask you some questions,' one said. 'Have you ever suffered from any mental disorder in the past?'

'Yes. A couple of years ago I was admitted to hospital with what was diagnosed as a persecution complex.'

'Why do you believe that you suffocated your grandfather?'

'The thought was inserted somehow into my mind by a traveller in the same compartment on a train journey.'

'You must come with us. If necessary we will summon the police. We are taking you to a hospital in Basingstoke where you will be treated for your illness. It is essential for you cooperate. Details of your work must remain undisclosed. We have been told that you worked on classified information in the naval department of your employers.'

After a phone call, an ambulance arrived and transported him to Park Prewett Hospital outside Basingstoke. A psychiatrist interviewed him and suggested that he undergo a course of electroconvulsive therapy. Norman's permission was requested in writing and, not knowing what was involved, Norman agreed. It was possible that Norman had a depressive illness of some sort at the time as well as schizophrenia, hence the reason for this treatment. It was something he dare not disclose to any non-medical person due to the derisory attitude of most of them to ECT. He did in fact read in a medical book that this treatment was not generally used for schizophrenia, only for depression. An anaesthetic was administered beforehand via an injection. This had the effect of making him lose consciousness, when then the therapy could be undergone. A cup of tea was offered afterwards. The persecutory thoughts that had invaded his mind quickly diminished and he made a rapid improvement.

On one occasion he happened to notice a beautiful reproduction of a painting by a French artist hanging from the hospital wall, and stood in front of it in admiration. It was called 'Mother and Child', and showed a female in a blue dress, sitting on a chair, holding a baby in her lap. On her lap was also a red rose. The mother and child both had blue eyes and this echoed the colour of her dress. A nurse happened to be present and Norman shared his admiration with her by remarking how much he admired it. She said a few words and then abruptly left. Somehow the painting reminded him of his own mother and an absent father, the absence signified by the red rose on the woman's lap.

Near the end of his stay in the hospital he had a discussion with the charge nurse about the future.

'Would you like to leave the hospital? You can stay if you wish. You might be able to find a female lover here. It might be difficult for you outside hospital.'

'I must leave as I have to continue my efforts to find a professional job,' Norman replied.

He had to make preparations for his departure from hospital. His first thoughts were of a financial nature, so he approached a local bank and asked to see the bank manager. Norman asked him if he could receive a loan, in response to which the manager asked if Norman had collateral. When Norman expressed unfamiliarity with the word 'collateral', the manager decided not to furnish a loan. Norman's 'collateral' was, as far as he was concerned, his educational qualifications; but these unfortunately were insufficient.

His financial problems were soon solved when Elliott's representative came to visit him in hospital. He stated that the company would continue paying him his full salary for three months to give him the opportunity of looking for a new job. He had asked whether Norman would be happy to return to work and be reunited with his colleagues. Whether his question was genuine or not was something Norman never found out.

Chapter Eight – Temporary Recovery

After some inquiries he found accommodation in a seedy hotel in London. He shared the room with a Scotsman who had long hair. His hairstyle was rather unfashionable then and did not become fashionable until the seventies. He tried to get Norman interested in the ordinary pleasures of life, beginning with a visit to a swimming bath. It was in spring and the pool was unheated. The coldness of the water made Norman gasp and he found it sharply exhilarating. He had no swimming trunks and just kept his underwear on. Nor could he swim, for that was the first time he had ventured into a swimming pool. They shared the same towel for drying themselves.

It seemed that his room-mate Jim was determined to broaden Norman's horizons. Jim took him in tow to a dance club in the West End. Norman was allowed to enter free of charge as Jim's guest. The dance floor was a seething mass of dancers and the temperature of the room was very high; there seemed to be no ventilation there. Jim left Norman at the bar and said he would try to find a couple of girls from the dance floor to keep them company. The song 'I heard it through the grapevine' resounded through the room, which appeared to be vibrating and shimmering in the heat. Norman was the only one who wasn't dancing and he felt a bit conspicuous at the bar on his own. The premises were so overheated that the sweat started to pour from him. Due partly to the heat and partly to the possible prospect of having to engage a female he did not know in conversation, he decided to leave, not waiting for Jim. The thought of meeting a female for the first time and engaging her in a steady flow of conversation was something that terrified him. If this situation had arisen he would not have had the confidence to deal with the female and from experience would expect them to make a quick exit from his presence.

After a couple of months had elapsed Norman's efforts to find employment bore fruit. He was taken on as a junior geophysical engineer by an oil exploration company.

'After an initial period of training for three months with us here, you will be sent to the field having a direct involvement in oil exploration. You will need a course of injections as there are various diseases you would be exposed to abroad that can be avoided through the injections.'

Norman was quite happy to accept the terms of agreement and started work the following week. In the few intervening days he managed to find accommodation in a hostel in Croydon, into which he moved immediately. The employer's training was very poor and was insufficient to meet Norman's needs. His superior, Nat, seemed to think that Norman should get any information he required from his fellow workers and should be able to make good relationships with them to achieve this cooperation. Nat gave him some basic information regarding geophysical maps on which he was to spend practically all his time on while employed by the company. Nothing new was explained or entrusted to him for the three months he stayed there, apart from one new aspect of the job, which necessitated him seeking help from a fellow worker. This other person made it clear he did not want to become involved and claimed it was Nat's responsibility to give the information.

He was only on good terms with one person there. That was a young employee called Paul, to whom Norman had given information on binary numbers. This had been gratefully received and Paul had been on friendly terms with him since. He often accompanied Norman to lunch at a local restaurant during the midday break. One such an occasion they were both seated in a restaurant and Norman confided in Paul that he thought a woman sitting at a table some distance away was admiring Paul.

'What makes you think that?' asked Paul.

'It's the expression on her face,' retorted Norman. 'She reminds me of a woman in a painting called "Mother and child".'

Paul did not relish the thought of her admiring him.

Soon it was time to discuss his future with the manager. Nat didn't pull his punches and claimed Norman was not making proper relationships with the rest of the staff. He urged Norman to sign a resignation form, otherwise he would be sacked. On looking back at this event, Norman felt that Nat had asked him to confess that he had schizophrenia – a medical name Norman was unfamiliar with – and reveal it in his letter of resignation. Norman had no option but to resign. He had saved a considerable amount from his salary over the three months he had been employed there. The weekly rent for the hostel was well within his means but the food was deplorable. The boiled potatoes inevitably tasted (and felt) like rocks. Tea was served from an urn that appeared not to be in a hygienic condition, as after breakfast Norman often retched. He made no effort to look for work at first, until his savings became more or less depleted, and would spend the time in his room reading library books.

He decided to return to writing his MSc thesis, as he had no commitments at that particular time. He turned to the problem of understanding the application of Riemann surfaces to the Corona Problem as written by Carleson. Within a few weeks Norman had overcome this problem and was able to replace this particular part of the paper by a more basic proof, but not as elegant as Carleson's. There remained one further problem near the end of Carleson's paper. Carleson referred to another paper of his near the end of his proof of the Corona Problem that was vital in his proof. It concerned a paper of his that showed how singular functions could be approximated by Blaschke products. The precise application was not clear to Norman, and he felt he had achieved something when he was able to show that certain types of outer functions could be approximated by Blaschke products as well and that this seemed vital to the proof of the Corona Problem. Perhaps Carleson had this in mind from the start.

He hired a typewriter and laboriously typed about seventy pages over a period of three weeks. He retained one copy, and the other two copies were sent to Aberdeen University, where they were bound for a small fee. Eventually they were accepted as suitable and he graduated MSc in absentia in December 1970. The long delay in submitting it was because Norman was not in the right frame of mind to continue where he had left off until that particular later time.

Finally, when his savings had considerably dwindled, he

applied for assistance from the social security, and was invited for an interview with a member of their staff for an assessment. The latter was annoyed at Norman and claimed that Norman, with his degree, should be in work. Norman had to admit he had mental health problems but was relieved when the official stated Norman would be awarded enough money to pay for his basic needs. He had never relied on the state before and detested being dependent on others for his survival.

Making a decision to avoid professional work, as that seemed beyond him, he finally succeeded in finding work as a sales invoice clerk. During the interview with the accountant, Norman was given the impression that there was a good possibility that there would be scope for accountancy training but that this aspect of the work would have to be home study. Norman felt that prospects there would be reasonable for him.

Unfortunately he was two weeks behind with his rent. He approached his landlord and requested that he be given the opportunity to pay the amount outstanding when he would receive his first month's salary. The landlord was unwilling to agree to this arrangement and demanded the outstanding amount as soon as possible. Norman's only option was to request an advance on his first month's salary, which he got with some reluctance from his employers.

In the hostel he became acquainted with a person who was a little eccentric, called David. One evening he met him outside the hostel and David took Norman into his confidence. David confided that his work colleagues treated him as an outsider and had very little to do with him. He confessed that he was paranoid. This seemed to be a picture of Norman himself, so Norman felt the reference might be directed at him. In any case Norman was in a stressful situation himself at work and had mentally deteriorated at his present job. On consulting his doctor, Norman was informed that the diagnosis that was made on him in Park Prewett Hospital was paranoid schizophrenia. He was also informed that David too was a patient of the doctor's, but the doctor made no reference to David's medical condition. This was after Norman had mentioned David's ambiguous comments about his paranoia to Norman.

He was still a keen fan of the cinema and one evening went to see *Ryan's Daughter* which was being shown in the West End. The film made a lasting impression on him as the heroine's name was Rosie and this name reminded him of his half-sister's name. The character played by John Mills seemed to be mentally disabled, and Norman felt that the situation in the film was a veiled reference to his own relationship with his sibling, Rosie. There seemed to be other aspects of the film that related to him as well and it was a delusion that would haunt him during the several relapses he was to encounter in the future.

On joining as a sales invoice clerk he was allocated to the senior clerk who was supposed to train him. Norman was seated alongside him but there was no instruction or explanation provided and the senior clerk continued doing his own work. This state of affairs continued for a month after which Norman had learnt nothing. In the end his superior asked him to sit at an empty table, where he remained for several hours. On looking back to the way things had developed there Norman blamed the lack of cooperation from his superiors on his poor personal hygiene. He had not developed a system for keeping his clothes regularly clean.

Eventually another invoice clerk was given the responsibility of training Norman. The work was straightforward apart from the telephone aspect related to it. The amount of telephone work was minimal but it was essential to keep a regular track of how much material had been supplied for various contracts. Norman decided to estimate these figures but should have confirmed this by telephone. His reluctance in using the telephone resulted in several contracts being under-invoiced, resulting in a loss of interest. Norman could see no way out and decided to look round for an alternative job.

Another factor that influenced Norman to look round for a different job was related to a contract with Rolls-Royce. Norman had unearthed an old contract made with this company that had been discontinued and left uninvoiced, so he decided to invoice them for the amount outstanding. A few days later he received a call from the manager of the manufacturing division in Scotland. Apparently Norman shouldn't have taken the initiative of invoicing Rolls-Royce. The manager had a thick Scottish accent and it was impossible to understand the drift of what he was saying. It transpired that a few weeks later Rolls-Royce crashed due to cash flow problems. Norman never discovered whether he had been partly responsible for this or not.

He had bought a book called *Schizophrenia* and a book on psychosomatic illness called *The Person in the Body* in a nearby medical bookshop. The latter had a section on the schizoid personality, describing a typical personality of that type as 'still waters run deep' as opposed to 'a bubbling brook in the spring-time' for the other extreme type of personality. The former book, however, was aimed at medical postgraduates, and Norman made heavy weather of it. From his understanding of his own illness he came to the conclusion that his illness was following a 'shift-like' course as described by the author, F J Fish. However, he had initially jumped to the conclusion that his illness had been wrongly diagnosed and was in actual fact periodic catatonia. This caused him a lot of distress, as Fish had asserted this illness resulted in permanent defect. Fish talked about loss of 'energy potential' in schizophrenia but this important concept was not clearly defined in his book. Norman felt that his illness at the age of thirteen, which had been diagnosed as rheumatic fever, followed by chorea at a later date, amounted in fact to catatonia. His two toes had become blue and discoloured at that time and this seemed to support his view of wrong diagnosis, as Fish claimed 'many catatonics had bluish extremities'.

He could also visualise himself as exhibiting, at that time, another catatonic symptom called 'psychological pillow'. This was a term describing the catatonic symptom of the patient having the head unsupported by the pillow underneath, and the patient maintaining himself in a rigid position several inches above. Norman's memory for that occasion might have been false, but even to the present day he can see it with what amounts to absolute clarity. It could amount to a type of memory falsification. Again he seemed to see himself as exhibiting stupor when examined by the doctor who diagnosed rheumatic fever.

Things came to a head in the hostel. One female whom he had eyed excessively barged into him as he was carrying his dinner on a tray towards the table. It seemed deliberate to him. He felt shattered at the incident and the food scattered on the floor, soiling the carpet. This strengthened his resolve to find new accommodation.

Finally he found a new job as a data control clerk, with the assumption that he would eventually study for actuarial qualifications. His salary for the position was at the maximum level, as his career was intended to become orientated towards actuarial work eventually. He had also been successful in finding a bedsitter in Lambeth. If only he had realised at that time that sex and material things shouldn't come first! His attitude should have been based on 'Rock of Ages':

> Nothing in my hand I bring.
> Simply to thy cross I cling;
> Naked, come to thee for dress;
> Helpless, look to thee for grace;
> Foul, I to the fountain fly;
> Wash me, Saviour, or I die.

The atmosphere in the insurance company head office where he worked as a data control clerk was quite relaxing. There was continuous pop music being played in the background, and this seemed to stimulate the workers to attack their work with vigour. It could be a trifle distracting, though, and on a number of occasions Norman found that his concentration was being affected to some extent, causing him to make mistakes. He felt his supervisor was unhappy with his quality of work as, on one occasion, the supervisor had asked him to check his output for that particular day again. Sure enough, Norman discovered he had made some errors, so he corrected them. This incident compelled him to resort to a policy of quality, not quantity. His attitude had been to maximise his output and this had not been appreciated. He had been doing twice the amount of work as the others in the same time, but unfortunately had committed a proportionate amount of inaccuracies.

After a couple of months had elapsed there an actuarial assistant tried to get Norman involved with some more advanced work. His explanation of the task was poor and Norman decided to ask another fellow worker for help. Sadly, he was unable to help much and Norman struggled with the work that had been allocated to him, until finally the actuarial assistant asked Norman to abandon the task and took over the work himself.

Soon afterwards a female supervisor allocated some work to his neighbour and placed some of the work on Norman's desk, advising Norman to ask his neighbour to explain how to proceed.

'Bitch, why didn't you explain it yourself?' Norman muttered, possibly within her earshot. He added to his neighbour, 'Can you explain what is involved to me, please?'

'No, I refuse to do that,' was his reply.

Norman had to resort to get clarification from someone more compliant. As he continued doing his allocated task he felt a lack of confidence in the way he was performing and he was relieved when it all came to an end.

At the end of his three months' probation he was summoned into the actuary's office.

'Are you ready to start your actuarial studies at college?' the latter asked.

'I am afraid I found the work that your assistant entrusted to me difficult to do. I am not really confident I can do it,' Norman replied.

'In that case you had better give way to someone else who can,' the actuary said.

Next day Norman decided to write to the insurance company giving in his notice. The following day again he decided to visit them to claim his outstanding wages and was met by stony silence from his workmates. He offered his supervisor a couple of pens which he had inadvertently taken home from work, as he felt his supervisor disapproved of such behaviour. It could have amounted to petty theft.

He decided to explore the possibility of a professional job through the Department of Employment for professional people. They took his details and within minutes they had found an interested employer and put him on the phone to them. Surprisingly it was Elliott Brothers, and they seemed quite interested. He did not want to reveal to them that he was a previous employer of theirs so he made the excuse that he had already found employment. The girl at the other end of the line seemed very exuberant and later he wondered if they had been giving him a second chance, or on the other hand expressing their disapproval in him.

The member of staff dealing with him in the employment exchange suggested he try a change in career and apply for a bookkeeping course that the Department of Employment organised twice yearly. He agreed to do this and was informed that the next course would start in September.

He was being seen regularly by a psychiatrist and a social worker attached to the Maudsley Hospital. The psychiatrist, Dr Noble, had arranged an appointment with him every fortnight, and tried to encourage him to keep taking regular medication. Unfortunately Norman found the drugs dispensed to him difficult to tolerate and had to discontinue using them. Norman was not very reliable at keeping appointments and missed a couple. At the next appointment Dr Noble kept him waiting alone in the appointment room for two hours after the other outpatients had gone. Eventually a member of staff came into the room and conducted him to the psychiatrist's room. That incident made Norman realise how important it was to keep appointments, and he made it a policy to be punctual in the future.

He had regular appointments with a social worker as well. She always dressed in a miniskirt and would sit provocatively in front of him displaying her thighs. Norman found her physical attractiveness almost overpowering. It was as if he were being hypnotised by her. He had to make a conscious effort to look away while conversing with her and this must have seemed an unusual mode of behaviour to her. Previous to Dr Noble's decision to keep him waiting he had missed an appointment with her and had turned up unannounced to her soon afterwards. She had been understanding about his unreliability and relinquished an hour of her time to talk to him. Norman had expressed concern about the lack of contact between him and the Department of Employment regarding the arrangement for starting his bookkeeping course, and the social worker suggested she phone them to clarify matters. She did this in his presence and was advised that Norman should approach them himself if he had any questions to ask about the arrangements.

Soon he started his bookkeeping course at Princeton College. The course covered English, arithmetic, typing and economics as well as bookkeeping itself. The English and arithmetic were superfluous in his estimation, as he already had all the necessary qualifications in these subjects. Emphasis was made on neatness and little on creativity. The bookkeeping was covered very laboriously over a period of six months, Norman feeling it could be condensed to a fortnight. After a few days in the college had elapsed, the head of the college summoned him to his office.

'What are you doing here with a Master's degree in Mathematics?' he bluntly asked Norman.

A female teacher was present, absorbed in her own work. Her presence made Norman more conscious of his frailties. The head had not the politeness to discuss the matter with Norman in private.

'I have had mental health issues in the past and this hampered my attempts to hold down a professional job,' he replied, flinching as he spoke. Afterwards he chided himself for not pointing out to the head that the course was meant to include people like him. Was it his fault that he was reduced to that position? Anyway the head seemed finally to acknowledge that he had a right to be attending the college.

The arithmetic teacher was called Miss Jones. She had an ordinary degree from Oxford, and Norman felt he had something in common with her for that very reason. She came in once in a miniskirt showing a black pair of briefs on bending down next to a desk. Norman expressed a chuckle to the nearest student and revealed to him how attractive he found her. Another member of the class obviously made his feelings more public and eventually Miss Jones had to reprimand him. The colour of her briefs seemed to have a special significance to Norman.

Another occurrence made him even more self-conscious in the classroom. Towards the end of the course, the bookkeeping teacher, Mr Costello uncovered a poster on the class wall underneath which another poster was hidden featuring two sumo wrestlers confronting each other, one being dark-skinned. That poster had cryptic comments displayed round the wrestlers, none of which made sense to Norman. He took it as a pointed reference to the relationship he had had with his previous landlord Sam. The people behind this vague implication were, as far as he could see it, MI5. They were showing him in their own oblique way that he had been unsuitable in his time of employment with Elliott Brothers, as he apparently had not revealed all his personal details to them. Admittedly he was very unstable mentally during this course and he could look back at this situation later on in life as a misunderstanding of events. However, as with all thoughts that affected him deeply, he retained some degree of belief in them on a permanent basis. Some part of his mind would never let completely go of them. Once a thought became deeply embedded in his mind during his worse moments, an element of belief remained even after recovery. It was never dismissed as complete fabrication.

Chapter Nine – Further Setback

Two weeks before the end of the course Norman felt he could not cope there any longer and sought help from his doctor. His doctor gave him a sick note covering two weeks which listed his illness as depression. Possibly Asian doctors group several illnesses together and refer to them all as 'depression'. Norman felt he had failed at the college as he had felt he had at university, and drew a parallel between them. There was an examination just before the end of the course in which he did not perform very well, having lost a vital two weeks due to being unwell. The college arranged an interview for him, which was for a book keeping vacancy. The interviewer asked him what his percentage in the final examination was, and when Norman answered the interviewer was a bit taken aback. Obviously he expected a better mark. Needless to say he was not offered the job.

He then had an interview at the employment exchange and was hopeful they would be successful in finding him suitable employment. They suggested a low-paid job with a charity, but that was completely out of the question for Norman as he would not be able to survive on the salary they offered. In any case he had previously had an interview with the charity involved and had been rejected for the post.

He decided to ignore the employment exchange's so-called 'assistance' and succeeded in finding a vacancy as assistant to the company secretary of a leasing company. Part of his work involved keeping the cash book up to date, so that some book-keeping was involved. The rest of his job mainly involved making leasing calculations for customers. After some thought, Norman was able to apply his mathematical knowledge to the leasing calculations to simplify the calculations, something that had not occurred to his employers as their knowledge of mathematics was limited. The majority of the leasing calculations could be made using a formula and verified by the use of a calculating machine. His employers were quite impressed.

The chairman and owner of the company was a liberal and invited Norman several times to accompany him for lunch at the National Liberal Club in Whitehall. On one occasion Norman tried to be adventuresome and ordered frogs' legs. The waiter did not recommend them so he opted for scampi and chips. On another occasion the chairman posed him the following mathematical problem:

If a donkey is tethered at the circumference of a circular field, how large should the rope be to allow it to graze on exactly half the field? Norman felt the problem had some bearing on him and asked whether he or the chairman was the donkey. This question was met with some indignation on the part of the chairman. He was so annoyed that Norman received no more invitations to lunch. Jeremy Thorpe was a director, and once signed Norman's pay cheque. Norman was tempted to keep the cheque as a souvenir but decided against it, as the monetary value of the cheque was more important to him. Norman's self-imposed restriction to his bed-sitting room when his mental problems again became severe – only leaving it to do his shopping – was what caused him to draw a comparison at a later time between himself and the donkey's situation.

The secretary was a young, attractive girl who was employed there during her school vacation. There was a weekly conference elsewhere that the staff attended, apart from Norman, who was left in charge of the empty offices. It was necessary for Norman to learn how to use the telephone keyboard in the secretary's absence so she made a hurried and half-hearted attempt to explain to him how to operate it. Her explanation was unsatisfactory and he had to ask for clarification from the office manager, with whom Norman failed to fare better.

On one afternoon when he was entrusted with the running of the office in the absence of the others he was unable to receive any incoming calls as he had interfered with the telephone keyboard, resulting in them being blocked. He dreaded those occasions when the offices were left in his care.

His work was accurate on the whole but one day he noticed an entry in the cash book that he didn't understand. He dealt with it incorrectly and within a few days the company secretary summoned him to his office and angrily demanded why he had made a wrong entry. It appeared that a client had not been credited with a leasing payment due to Norman's mistake, and was in the office in person to clarify things. The company secretary was livid.

Eventually the stress related to the job and that incident in particular tipped him over the edge and he became seriously ill. The fact that he was not on medication did not help; he was to find out later that he needed to take medication for life; he was unaware of this fact then. He decided he could not face his employers any more and that he had let them down. Therefore he gave his notice in writing by post, as he was unable to discuss matters with them face to face.

Soon his health deteriorated even further, and his mental symptoms were accompanied by physical symptoms as well. One evening he experienced severe burning pains running through his body that convinced him that he was being poisoned. There seemed no other logical explanation for it all. He feared that jealous neighbours resented the fact that he was existing on benefits while they had to work, and were making this known to him in no uncertain fashion. He felt he was being tested to see how much he could bear.

Eventually he had to seek help and presented himself with his problems at the Maudsley, desperate for help. He was seen by a young oriental nurse.

'Nip off and get me a psychiatrist, Nippon,' Norman said.

'I am not Japanese. I come from Thailand. Wait here until I return.'

Eventually she did return with the duty psychiatrist who, after interviewing Norman, had no hesitation in admitting him as an inpatient there and then, where he remained for six months. His thinking was bizarre. An example of his flawed reasoning was that he associated the re-released song 'Sixteen Tons' with the character Brick in *Cat on a Hot Tin Roof*. When asked to clarify this he said his problems were like heavy weights under which he was burdened (tons), and felt Brick (Brixton) had a similar problem through possible illicit sex, as Norman himself had. Norman had always enjoyed Tennessee Williams, finding his style so beautiful. He liked to draw a connection with one of his characters and himself. When asked what Brick's problem was, he replied that his problem was being married and having a wife to placate with under the situation he found himself in. The suggestion made by Norman was that he, himself, did not have a wife to please, so in a sense had differences as well as similarities regarding Brick.

Many of the inpatients in his ward were professional people. One patient was even a consultant psychiatrist. Another patient, called Tom, had been taken ill during his MA studies on the history of art. He often invited Norman to play a relaxing game of snooker with him. Tom's snooker was appalling but Tom still seemed to release some inward tension through this sport.

The female ward and the male ward shared a common lounge. That was where he made the acquaintance of a Greek girl called Chrisanthe. She was a second year student in science who first caught his attention as she was blithely walking up and down the lounge reciting Homer's *Odyssey* from a book that she held in her hands. Her affectionate and sweet nature had him spellbound but he dare not show his feelings to her. He would feel jealous if he saw her converse with anyone else. He felt he could not share her with anyone else. She played chess with him on several occasions but was hopeless at the game. She seemed to find it relaxing and enjoyable despite her poor standard of play. Instead of recovering she seemed to deteriorate, and at one point begged Norman to help her. He did not want to show her how fond he was of her and just replied that he was sorry she was unwell. Her family and two sisters visited her regularly and he used to observe her reaction to her family's presence. Her family included a young boy to whom she seemed to react unfavourably. Norman wondered if the boy could have been her son but he never found out. It seemed to Norman that she confided in him in order to lead him on.

After a period of about three months in hospital the psychiatrist advised him to look for employment. A hospital aptitude test was arranged for him to determine whether office work would be suitable for him. He achieved a high percentage in it, and the next step was to get him involved doing clerical work in hospital as a preparation for eventual work outside. Several weeks were spent on these tasks. They went well, apart from one occasion when Norman used his own initiative on a task and incurred the annoyance of the nurse who was supervising the work. It was impossible to start on the task afresh as the original documents involved had been destroyed. The nurse was very annoyed, claiming that the work was not just a diversion for Norman to familiarise himself with office work, but an important and essential task for assisting in the administration of the hospital.

Through the employment exchange he was successful in finding work with a travel agency as an accounts assistant. The accountant was not very skilled at instructing Norman, and as a result the latter was only entrusted with simple chores. A considerable part of the working day was spent in idleness, reading a paper to while away the time. The situation was tense. The room in which he worked was occupied by the accountant's secretary, as well as by the accountant himself. There was little conversation between the three, as the accountant seemed very engrossed in his work. The secretary confided in Norman that she would soon be returning to her native country, Australia, to a farm that was very isolated. She expressed concern that she might not be able to find a boyfriend in such a remote area. Norman tried to console her but his words did not seem to have the desired effect on her. She was not a very attractive girl and her problem was very real. Norman felt that her main problem was her inadequate appearance and hoped she didn't detect this view in his dealings with her in general.

He had to regularly consult various travel assistants in the premises about their transactions and found this task very stressful. He was uncertain if he should be doing this, thinking that it was unnecessary, and that there might be some other approach to finding the information without having to resort to asking them individually. He felt they resented his interference as they gave the impression of being very engrossed in their work. One of them had a Bible in her desk drawer and Norman noticed her reading it on several occasions. He felt closer to her than with any of the rest of the staff; she reminded him of his family, who were all Christians at this time. There was a tranquillity about her that impressed him. She always greeted him with a benign smile.

He was still a hospital inpatient as the psychiatrists felt that the transition to work would be more controlled if he remained in the hospital for the first few months of work. However, his period of work soon came to an end.

'I think we had better call it a day!' the accountant snapped at him.

'Do you mean you want me to give in my notice?' Norman replied, shocked at how the accountant had expressed himself.

'Yes,' the accountant responded, tersely.

It was with a certain amount of relief that Norman discussed his position at work with the manager. The manager stated that the accountant was not the best of instructors. This was of some consolation to Norman, who had felt he was to blame for not coping with the work successfully. The manager said he would be pleased to furnish Norman with a reference in the future if need be. On his last day of work and just before his departure from the office, Norman experienced very bitter feelings about the accountant's failure to train him to do his job effectively. He took the opportunity when the office was empty to remove some of the accountant's documents and flush them down the toilet. He had a feeling of satisfaction at this decision, and stalked out of the offices for the last time, saying goodbye only to the manager. His colleagues appeared absorbed in their work as he went off. There was a heavy downpour as he exited the travel agency, and this somehow reminded him of nuclear fallout. He felt as if some catastrophe had materialised out of the blue. He made his way dejectedly back to his bed-sitting room, having been discharged from hospital at this time.

He had to rely on assistance from the employment exchange to find alternative employment. On one occasion his name was announced to see a member of the department's staff and he hopefully went to the cubicle where the latter was sitting with a pocket watch in her hand.

'What is your name?' she asked.

Norman hesitated at the strangeness of the remark, as his name had just been announced. He felt bewildered. After some further hesitation on Norman's part, he stated his name. The girl made a note on a piece of paper.

'Sorry, we have nothing for you,' she replied.

It was many years afterwards that Norman came to the realisation that she had been timing his response speed, and that she had judged him unsatisfactory. This had been a degrading procedure for him; when the realisation occurred to him he felt furious at his treatment. However, he returned to the employment exchange on a later date and was advised that there was a vacancy for a filing clerk and was advised to apply for it. This he did, and was interviewed and accepted by the interviewer. The location was next to Westminster Abbey – a firm of solicitors.

On his first day he was ushered into a basement room and introduced to the person whom he was replacing. This person was involved with the legal side of the business and the filing was only a minor part of his duties. He was due to retire in two weeks. His name was Wilfred.

'I am just in the process of completing a reduction in the amount of files stored here,' Wilfred said, continuing, 'I have created a considerable amount of free space that you will find useful. In the meantime, as I continue with this task, you can apply yourself to reading some of the material available here, until I have time to devote to your training.'

'Thank you. I have always been an admirer of Agatha Christie and will read this book that she has written: *The Murder of Roger Ackroyd*.'

'You will not be involved in any of the legal work,' Wilfred said. 'Your task will be to deal with the filing only.'

It transpired from trivial conversation exchanged between the two of them that Wilfred had a grandson who had recently entered university. Norman admitted that he had a degree in mathematics. Norman's position in life made him feel inadequate, as Wilfred seemed to have high aspirations for his grandson. Another reason for Norman's feelings was that filing required only a little intelligence, although his starting salary was very generous. This situation would make him uneasy, as other staff there did more demanding work and were not paid any more than him.

When Wilfred finally left, Norman was in sole control of the filing. The filing was composed of two separate systems and Norman was asked to combine both into one. This he did, having had to apply some amount of intelligence to that task, which took two weeks to complete. It gave him satisfaction that he had completed this correctly.

He found that very little time was necessary to do the filing. A solicitor might phone him and require a file. Norman would then retrieve the file from the shelves and deliver it to the person who requested it. Requests for files only occurred a few times a day only, creating a considerable amount of free time for Norman – a situation he was uneasy about. He felt he was paid for doing nothing. He would buy a newspaper and would spend a lot of his time in his office reading it from first page to last, leaving nothing out. He received luncheon vouchers, which contributed towards the cost of his meals. He felt rather uncomfortable visiting the local restaurants, preferring not to give tips and therefore selecting self-service restaurants. He tried several and in the end found one that seemed ideal, the staff there being friendly.

The staff, and the solicitors themselves, were reasonably friendly and there was one female solicitor in particular called Christine whom Norman found devastatingly attractive. He cringed with embarrassment when he received a smile from her direction. He hated interacting with her in any way as he felt he would betray his feelings for her and that she would find them repulsive. She did not require Norman's help much and that state of affairs suited him, as his fondness for her was too overpowering for him.

One of the staff, called Ron, was a messenger for the solicitors' firm. The manager had suggested that the staff become familiar with each other's work in order to temporarily replace a member who might be on holiday. Norman accompanied Ron several times on his messenger duties in order to familiarise himself with Ron's work. This involved delivering letters to the House of Commons and to 10 Downing Street. Norman was so unhappy with his idleness that he suggested to Ron that he take over some of Ron's messenger duties. Ron was quite happy with this suggestion. When Norman visited the House of Commons to deliver his letters he found the people in the room where he had been instructed to leave his letters very uncommunicative. They would be engrossed in reading newspapers and would not even raise their heads to say hello. Eventually Norman was asked to deliver the documents to another part of the House of Commons, and this involved taking a lift to another floor. The lift attendant never conversed with Norman and remained surly and morose.

Finally, the circumstances surrounding his place of employment, the fact that people might despise him for not being successful in finding a professional job, and a few mistakes he had made that he magnified enormously, made Norman decide to leave his job. He left suddenly without giving in his notice and with three weeks' wages owing to him. He did not communicate with them about this and lost further contact with them. He was seriously ill again and entertained strange beliefs about those around him. He felt bitter at the staff, feeling that they had contributed to his present situation. His attitude should have been as summed up in Luke:

> If you love those who love you, what credit is that to you? Even sinners love those who love them... But love your enemies, do good to them, and lend to them without expecting to get anything back.

He remained confined to his room from that point onwards and was so disillusioned about his experiences at work that he made no effort to look for alternative employment. Deterioration in his mental health increased until he reached the stage where he could not depend on his senses any more. He seemed more acutely aware of noises that became more and more unreal to him. In particular he seemed to hear the frequent aeroplanes that passed overhead on their way to Heathrow differently. To him, the engines seemed to be echoing like trumpets the snatches of tunes that would sometimes flit through his head. The tunes did not seem to originate within him but from the aeroplanes flying overhead. His interpretation of the situation was that his mind was being experimented upon by the medical authorities, who were investigating the complexity of the human mind and using him as a guinea pig.

Chapter Ten – Further Deterioration

He remained confined to his room for several months while his health deteriorated further. His mother occasionally visited him but he rejected all offers of help, having made the decision not to visit his doctor or psychiatrist again. They were part of the experiment and were colluding in it. In the end he felt practically everyone were involved in the 'experiment'. He suffered from severe pains in his chest, which he thought the landlord was responsible for, through poisoning his water supply. He decided on one occasion to ask the lady living underneath him to give him a glass of water, which she did. It would have fitted the situation perfectly if she had replied to remind him that:

> Then the righteous will answer him, 'Lord, when did we see you hungry and feed you, or thirsty and give you something to drink? When did we see you a stranger and invite you in or needing clothes and clothe you? When did we see you sick or in prison to visit you?' The king will reply, 'I tell you the truth, whatever you did for one of the least of these brothers of mine, you did for me.'

Eventually he could bear no more and lashed out indirectly at the landlord by breaking the front door and several windows. The matter had evidently been reported to the police, as he found two policemen on his doorstep within a short time. They questioned him about the damage to the property and asked if he was responsible for it. Norman did not deny it and admitted to it. The sergeant had a strong resemblance to a sergeant in the television series *Z-Cars* and this suggested to Norman that somehow the television was involved. As a result he did not realise the gravity of the situation. The authorities came to the decision to transfer him to hospital, as a psychiatrist diagnosed mental health problems.

On admission to the hospital he was immediately confined to bed. He was supplied with pyjamas that were unfortunately too tight for him, with the result that a certain part of his body was embarrassingly exposed. Requesting other pyjamas from a nurse, he was met with sarcasm from her. Norman interpreted this reaction as being a continuation of the plot he still believed was in operation. She did offer him another set of pyjamas that were fortunately a better fit. The incident seemed to suggest to him that deliberate attention was being focussed on his genitals due to his illicit relations in the past. He felt that he was under the microscope and that he was the centre of attraction there. He feared to join the other patients for tea, as he felt they disapproved of his past sexual behaviour. He was advised to undergo regular injections of a drug called depixol to improve his condition. The choice of administering a drug by injection rather than orally was because he would be less likely to discontinue taking it, as he would not have to be relied on to take it orally.

There was quite an active programme of occupational therapy in the hospital, and Norman was encouraged to take part. Scrabble was a pursuit Norman found stimulating and he was often invited by other patients to make up a group in order to play it. He prided himself in having an adequate vocabulary to equip him to play reasonably well at it. However, the play was dominated by another player who gave the game an excessive amount of thought. There would occasionally be criticism of the amount of thought this player would apply to the games. Some players found his slowness annoying, but it seemed to pay dividends for him as he invariably came first.

A class was held by two female occupational therapists that involved various interests. Once they discussed the history of art and provided a slide show of various well-known paintings. A slide of a painting by L S Lowry caught Norman's imagination as the depiction of human figures was a reminder of the lack of humanity he had experienced in people. Sadly, he found all the activities there distasteful. This was the wrong attitude, and may have stemmed from his past passion for mathematics, which he found irreplaceable. Despite this, he was to develop an attraction for the history of art in later life and regretted not taking it up at this earlier stage. He did not apply himself fully to the therapy, finding no interest in the activities. Somehow they did not seem to be stimulating enough for him. His future social life might have turned out differently if he had taken up some of the activities at that particular time.

'Have you had any interests in the past?' asked a nurse once to him.

'Not really,' he replied, adding as an afterthought, 'apart from swimming, which interested me for a time several years ago. I took some swimming lessons and can do the breaststroke, although I am not really very proficient at it. I decided to learn after being invited by a fellow Scotsman to accompany him to a local swimming baths a few years ago.'

'We can arrange to take a group to the local swimming baths free of charge if you would be interested,' she replied. 'We could arrange to go there once a week. You would be accompanied by other patients, some who would be merely spectators.'

'Thank you for taking so much interest in me. I would be quite happy to go with you all.'

Regular visits to the baths were made. Norman did get a certain amount of enjoyment from these trips but was keenly aware that he was a very poor swimmer in comparison to the other swimmers in the baths. He was slightly overweight at that time and was conscious of his pot belly. His excess weight might have contributed to his feeble attempts at swimming. There was one female in the group, with whom he had made eye contact with several times before and whom he had found attractive. He had no opportunity to talk to her as another male patient had appeared to have captivated her attention. Norman felt cheated and disappointed when he saw them in animated conversation with one another.

The few weeks before his discharge he attended the hospital day centre to make a proper transition to life outside hospital. Routine work was provided there but it was of a repetitive nature. It was mainly assembly work and Norman found it very boring. However he persisted until he was discharged from hospital, having been an inpatient there for six weeks. Visits to the day centre continued after discharge. The workers received a small amount of money to encourage them to continue coming. It was all for their own benefit.

Having had to leave his previous bedsitter due to being admitted into hospital, he now had to find accommodation on his discharge from hospital. He fortunately discovered another bedsitter through an employment agency. He moved in immediately he was discharged from hospital. His total possessions could all be crammed into a single suitcase. The cooking facilities were minimal and it would be impossible to create a culinary masterpiece with what was provided. In any case, Norman did not cook appetising meals for himself, being content to heat up a tin of soup or something similar for his meal. He had never experimented in cooking nice meals and would continue in that vein for many years. The rent was very reasonable – just five pounds a week. It was collected monthly by the landlady, who came to collect it personally every four weeks. She would always bring up the subject of the weather, never entertaining any other type of conversation. She probably felt embarrassed, as Norman usually answered the door in his pyjamas, spending the whole day confined to bed. He was barely on speaking terms with the other residents.

Norman was not successful in making close relationships. He maintained himself at a distance, not giving himself emotionally to others. He was on reasonable terms with the other outpatients but felt emptiness within himself when he observed others making friends. He regarded himself as undeserving of friendship and incapable of responding in a genuine and warm way to others. In the late afternoon, on his way home from the day centre, he was accompanied by another outpatient who admitted he was a spastic. He seemed quite capable of managing his own affairs but there was no conversation in him. Norman found the journeys testing and was not a very good conversationalist himself. He confided in a therapist, who tried to put him at his ease.

He still resolved to make an attempt to be in regular employment, mainly for the financial security that it would bring. He was now resigned to the sad position that he would never be able to work in a professional capacity. This attitude always came to prominence during the periods he was employed doing clerical work, where he always felt unfulfilled due to his belief that the type of work was menial. He was determined to continue making an effort to remain in employment, having been encouraged to do so by psychiatrists in the past. He felt their main motive was to prevent him from dwelling on his own situation excessively, and that employment could divert him from those destructive thoughts.

He found employment as a data control clerk quite soon afterwards. His poor work record and his difficulty in finding suitable references proved a stumbling block for him. He had to resort to filling in the application form falsely, in such a way that it appeared he had been with his previous employer for several years, whereas in fact he had only been employed by them for three months. He was concerned about the outcome when his present employers would take up references with his previous employer. He found one aspect of the work difficult, and on seeking assistance from the female supervisor he was snapped at and told she was too busy. This deterred him from seeking any more information from her. He was nervous about using the phone and tried to avoid answering it when possible. He was not confident enough about doing his general work to answer related problems on the phone. He decided to confide in the occupational therapists, who advised him to discuss his aversion for the phone with his manager.

This he did, and found the discussion uncomfortable as the female supervisor was present as well. Norman was told that another member of staff would be quite happy to respond to phone calls when necessary. He derived little comfort from this arrangement, feeling dissatisfied with it as it drew attention to his shortcomings. He regretted having brought the subject up in the first place with his employer. The outcome of his employers taking up references, coupled with his uncertainty about doing his work correctly, made him decide to give in his notice after being there for only three weeks. He did not have the courage to do this face to face but decided on a letter of resignation through the post.

After Norman had been unemployed for a few weeks, the employment officer suggested a complete change of career. He drew Norman's attention to a company called Remploy, who were supported by the government to enable them to employ people who were registered as disabled. It was essential that

Norman be registered disabled first, and to Norman's surprise his doctor was willing to cooperate and agree to his registration. The wages that Remploy offered for assembly work were comparable to those Norman had received through office work in the past. The employment officer was present at the interview and had agreed to supply a reference. The interview went well and Norman was hired as an assembler.

The work involved assembling various objects such as lamps from their component parts. Emphasis was placed on speed, and a bonus was offered for the completion of more lamps than an average within a certain time range. Norman's speed was just above average and his bonus was minimal. Some of his co-workers, although disabled, were very competent at their jobs, and received a good bonus. Norman found the work repetitive and very tedious. An aspect of the work that caused him to become perturbed was that all of the workers seemed to be responsible for finding their own boxes into which the completed lamps and other objects should be placed. Sometimes there were so many empty boxes available that they were piled up in vast quantities at the back of the factory floor; at other times there would be none available.

Initially he sat next to a young girl called Tina, with whom he did not converse at all. Everyone continued to be engrossed in their work and there was no conversation, as there was in offices. The only opportunity for that came during the two ten-minute tea breaks, but Norman would always wait for someone to talk to him first and initiate a conversation. There was a half-hour dinner break and the dinner was consumed in a canteen. The portions were rather small but the prices were subsidised and very reasonable. Norman always hoped that his portion of boiled potatoes would be adequate, and this thought must have been transparent on his face, as the dinner assistant once complained to her companion that Norman was dissatisfied with the portion that had been allocated to him, although Norman had not revealed his thoughts in words. This experience unsettled him as he felt his thoughts might be apparent from his facial expression.

'Did you see the expression on his face? We have only a

limited amount of potatoes to go round. I am not being deliberately mean. What does he expect?'

As a result of this experience, Norman decided to conceal his expression in that situation in the future. He usually sat alone at dinner and once made eye contact with an attractive young girl on crutches. He tried to catch her eye again repeatedly and on numerous occasions but she failed to respond and never looked in his direction again. These occurrences were instrumental in eroding his self-confidence. One of the dinner assistants had blue eyes that struck Norman as being particularly beautiful, and they would often make eye contact as Norman queued up to be served. Sadly for him, a collection that dashed his hopes was made in the factory.

'Who is the collection for?' he asked, after making a modest contribution.

'It is for Angela's impending wedding,' was the reply. Angela was the girl with the beautiful blue eyes that had captivated Norman. The thought came to him that if he had made an effort to make her acquaintance she might be marrying him now and not someone else.

One of Norman's visits to his sister ended in tragedy soon afterwards. He was running to catch a moving bus on his way home when he fell off the platform onto the road and seriously damaged his hand. It was diagnosed by the doctor as a broken hand and his arm was put in a sling. The doctor said that with that type of injury a plaster would not be recommended. He received a doctor's certificate to be absent from work for three weeks until the hand healed. That was Norman's only absence, but it served to draw his attention to the boredom he had felt at work; he felt happy and relieved during the three weeks off work and this incident helped to focus on his dissatisfaction at his work as an assembler. One day at work the shortage of boxes to accommodate his assembled objects was so severe that the assembled lamps overflowed all over his desk onto the floor. Norman could not cope any more and decided to post a letter of resignation when he arrived home that evening. He had been there for one and a half years. He had been wise during that period at work and had succeeded in saving a considerable amount of money. His savings were fairly adequate at that time in his life.

'Be content with your pay,' uttered John the Baptist to those around him. The salary Norman received was adequate for the work he did.

Norman made a decision at that time not to work again. He was very disillusioned about his past employment and decided he could not cope with work again. He was content with the money supplied from the social security due to his circumstances in life.

He discovered a Chinese takeaway nearby and started to go there regularly, as he found their food enjoyable and very different from English food. Eventually he started visiting it several times a week, selecting several portions on each visit. He became concerned about his weight, as he appeared to increase his weight by about half a stone a fortnight. Finally his weight escalated to seventeen stones. His clothes became too tight for him and would often split at the seams. He found it difficult to find clothes that would fit, especially pyjamas. He discontinued his visits to the takeaway and with determination he restricted his calorific intake to 1,200 calories a day. This had a pronounced effect and he began losing weight consistently.

One day about that time his mother related to him the sad fact that her husband, Harry, had been diagnosed as having lung cancer. Harry had been a regular cigarette smoker all his life. He was given at most six months to live. This sentence made him come to the decision to stop smoking immediately. Norman expressed sympathy for him, but at the same time was pleased that the mental cruelty that Harry had inflicted on his mother would come to an end; she would soon be free of him. She announced this sentiment verbally to him. 'The Lord took him away because He knew I could only bear so much.'

She meant a spiritual, as well as physical, death. Norman never saw Harry in the flesh again, although Norman's sister, Ann, who was a Christian, visited him and comforted him during a brief stay in hospital. He was discharged, and on one occasion, according to Norman's mother, the pain was so severe that he continually screamed. Painkilling drugs were administered to him, but he died within six weeks, not six months. Norman's mother now had freedom that she had never experienced before. She was now financially secure, having received a lump sum and a pension from Harry's employers.

Chapter Eleven – Family Changes

Norman's mother, Nora, had decided to visit Bayble, the place of her birth, some time before her husband's death. To this end she had accumulated £200 over quite a long period, but when Harry died she could visit Bayble without being concerned about the financial aspect of the visit.

'Ann and Iain are accompanying me,' she said. 'You are welcome to come too, Norman. You would love to renew your acquaintance with the cliffs below which you spent so many happy hours fishing. Your old school friends would be delighted to see you again. Seeing the village and the surrounding country-side would be a wonderful experience for you as well.'

'I feel I have accomplished so little in my life,' Norman told her. 'I feel embarrassed about my mental health problems. I went to university and never used my degrees. I am unemployed... what would my response be if they asked me what my occupation was? I have never had a girlfriend, and never even took a lady friend out to the cinema or theatre; nor have I ever taken a girl out for a meal. I would have to reveal my present circumstances to those people and I feel too conscious about my past failures. I cannot accompany you for those reasons.'

'These reasons aren't valid ones,' his mother replied. 'Your acquaintances up there would not judge you for circumstances that are not your fault.'

Norman was determined not to go, as he lacked the courage to face those he formerly knew, with so little to boast about. The day came when they all – excluding Norman – boarded a taxi and made their way to the station, from which they took a train to Inverness and a ferry to the island they intended visiting. Norman jokingly urged Iain, Norman's half-brother, not to return home without a Lewis girl in tow.

After they left Norman put the finishing touches to his diet, having lost five stones over a period of six months. He was now a modest eleven stones in weight. He was never to become excessively overweight again, and he became more conscious of the variety of food that was available in the supermarkets. He would occasionally make an effort to cook a pleasant meal, as he had become more aware of the different food on the shelves in the shops through his scrutiny of their calorific content.

His family returned from Lewis after a very enjoyable holiday there. They had stayed at a hotel in the town of Stornoway and were very enthusiastic about the quality of the meals they had received there. A past neighbour of theirs had put his car at their disposal and during their stay had driven them round the island. Norman's mother related how they had arrived on the outskirts of Bayble for the first time after a bus journey from town. Walking from the bus stop they noticed someone they recognised and he greeted them, welcomed them to his home, and his wife provided a lovely meal for them. They were warmly welcomed by all their old neighbours. The house Norman had been brought up in lay in ruins and it was with sadness that they viewed it. Part of the roof had collapsed and it had been uninhabited for many years. Most of the people that they regarded as elderly were now dead.

'Your acquaintances in Bayble all asked for you, Norman,' his mother stated, and added, 'it was the best holiday we've ever had, and the weather was perfect for the duration of our stay.'

'I regret not accompanying you, as the trip seemed so pleasant for you all,' Norman answered. He felt a great deal of nostalgia during the recounting of the holiday they had spent in the most familiar place on earth to him.

Norman would visit his mother, sister and half-brother at their home every weekend and would stay there for the duration of the weekend. He had a habit of teasing his mother that she found objectionable. He would pull faces at her out of devilment but mainly because he was in a joyful mood. She would respond by throwing objects at him, frequently missing. This would be followed by a long period of sulky silence that Norman found difficult to bear. His frequent disagreements and disputes with his mother started from this time. Previously they had never had an argument during their relationship. The arguments would be about trivial things, and there used to be a long pregnant silence following it. Norman was probably at fault due to the effect of his illness upon him, resulting in bizarre behaviour towards his mother.

The three of them were devout Christians and they regularly attended a Pentecostal church. Norman looked on their belief with derision and used to mock them when they talked in tongues. Ann was particularly filled with the Holy Spirit, and Norman did not understand the gift of talking in tongues, which he thought was empty babbling. He would refuse to sit at the table during a meal while his mother blessed the food, and this caused bitter arguments between them. Norman didn't understand that we should thank God for His love for us by providing us with food and many other things we need. Norman's sister, Ann, had made several Christian friends through her visits to church. She was particularly close to a person with a similar name called Anne. Anne and Ann would frequently talk in tongues and Norman couldn't bear this. This behaviour served to intensify Norman's antagonism to Christianity and all that it stood for. Ann was having mental health problems at this time, and on several occasions she had to summon her pastor to pray for her in her home. The pastor's attitude was that the problem that had to be faced by her was not that she had mental health problems but that her brother was an atheist. Norman laughed out loud at this.

'The fool says in his heart "there is no God".'

Having been advised by his mother to apply for a council flat two years previously, he was surprised to receive a letter from the council suggesting he view a vacant flat. Unfortunately the postcode on the letter was incorrect, and this resulted in Norman receiving the letter after the date specified for viewing. Within three weeks another letter was delivered to Norman inviting him to view a flat in Angell Town, Brixton. Responding to the letter, Norman appeared for the viewing and discussed the vacant flat with a member of the council. Norman expressed concern at the locality of the flat as there had been a programme recently on television called *Angell Town*, which highlighted the crime in that area. The response from the housing officer was that the programme exaggerated the problems in that area. On inspecting the flat, Norman found it adequate and decided to accept the offer and stated he would move there in three weeks.

Norman was in the fortunate position that he had sufficient savings to cover the cost of supplying his flat with furniture. Some of the furniture he chose to buy was from a store near his mother's flat, so he decided to store it in her flat and arrange the removal at a future date. In the meantime he bought a cooker and fridge-freezer in Brixton. He arranged to have the rooms carpeted before he moved in properly. His sister recommended a removal firm, the owner of which was a Christian she knew. The firm delivered the furniture for a very competitive rate.

A few weeks after moving in he awoke one morning to hear a repetitive sound whose source initially baffled him. To his horror he detected a leak in his ceiling, and the rain was steadily dripping into his living room from the ceiling. He reported it immediately to the neighbourhood office, where he was informed that it would be dealt with within six weeks. After a long delay a council official came to inspect it and explained that the felt along the drains had cracked and was letting in water. He was pessimistic about when it would be eventually repaired, stating that it wasn't urgent. The carpet would get soaked whenever it rained and the dampness spread over the entire living room floor.

As the leaks were along the edge of the ceiling, Norman decided to discover if his neighbour had the same problem with her ceiling as he had. She showed Norman in and, sure enough, her kitchen was leaking. She introduced herself as being a primary school teacher. She was black and quite attractive in appearance. She confided in him that she had reported the leaks to the council but that she had had no response from them thus far. After numerous visits to the neighbourhood office, Norman decided to go in person to the roofing manager in the local depot. The manager claimed that he had attempted to contact Norman twice by leaving personally delivered letters to his flat for him and that there had been no response from him. Despite Norman's claims that he had never received the alleged letters, the manager appeared not to believe him. The manager gave Norman some forms to deliver to the neighbourhood office to speed up the repair process, and when Norman presented them to the neighbourhood officer he was met with a torrent of abuse from him. The repair was finally completed about a year after it had been reported.

It was with concern that Norman was informed that his sister had been admitted to a general hospital. On visiting her with his mother they discovered that she had been diagnosed as having a mobility problem called Guillain-Barré syndrome. The fact that it had remained misdiagnosed for some time prevented her from receiving the correct treatment initially, with the result that she incurred a permanent mobility problem. She coped with it bravely, however, and although initially she had to rely on a walking frame, she was able to discard it after a short period of time. Her mother always remarked on his sister's reliance on God to pull her through that illness.

Ann, together with Norman's mother, used to visit Norman for a few hours every Thursday. This arrangement continued over a period of a few years until Ann's visits became shorter and shorter, and eventually consisted of a duration of about twenty minutes only. Once, when she was expected, she didn't make an appearance and, concerned for her welfare, Norman decided to phone her to investigate the reason for her absence. It transpired that she had felt tired. From that time she became unreliable at keeping appointments. Nora, Norman's mother, often prepared meals for her family, including Ann. Ann sometimes didn't put in an appearance and failed to notify Nora by telephone when she had decided not to come. As a result the food and its preparation were often wasted. Nora found her daughter's behaviour difficult to tolerate and was very concerned about her mental state. It was all understandable, as Ann's behaviour was a result of her mental health problems. Ann's best friend, Anne, then died of cancer. Ann's pastor, who had been so supportive towards her, died quite soon afterwards from cancer. This was followed by the death of other friends, so that in the end Ann was deprived of most of the people who had been close to her.

At that time Norman longed to find a female friend with whom he could develop a close relationship before age finally destroyed his dreams. He was confined to his flat all day and had no opportunity to meet people. In the end, in frustration, he decided to correspond with a female, who was about twenty – a considerable amount of years younger than him – whom he contacted through a dating agency. They exchanged a few letters and she supplied him with a photograph. She looked rather obese and this deterred him. He was reluctant to show any profound interest in her via his correspondence in case this would deter her from continuing the relationship. A well-known Irish song came to his mind at that point.

> At the crossroads fair, I'll be surely there
> And I'll dress in my Sunday clothes,
> And I'll try sheep's eyes, and deludhering lies
> On the heart of the nut-brown rose.
>
> No pipe I'll smoke, no horse I'll yoke
> Though with rust my plow turns brown –
> Till a smiling bride by my own fireside
> Sits the star of the County Down.

She may possibly have been Irish, but his efforts to win her heart were very passive and indirect, as implied by the second half of the lines quoted here. In her third letter to him she intimated that she had been with her boyfriend that week. This sounded to Norman as if he had been replaced by another whom she preferred to him, so he decided to bring the correspondence to an end. This episode did little for his self-confidence.

He was not very experimental with his meals, and they were basic affairs. As he had an electric oven he was encouraged to try out some recipes while making sure that their calorific value was reasonably low. This excluded quite a lot of products since he was determined to maintain his weight at eleven stones. He hoped his new figure would make him more appealing to the opposite sex. It may have, but he lacked the courage to take the initiative, and he did not go out actively seeking a girlfriend. He felt he had very little to offer, being jobless and without money or a car, so he continued his isolated existence.

Chapter Twelve – Some Setbacks

Life remained the same for many years until seven years later, when Norman developed a breakdown for no apparent reason. The episode started with worrying thoughts that prevented him from obtaining any sleep for three days in succession. His weakness and tiredness resulted in the development of delusions in his mind regarding his MSc. He felt that his own contributions to his MSc had had military applications, which had been hidden from him by MI5. The research by Lennart Carleson that comprised the bulk of his MSc had been supported by a grant from the US Airforce. This was a definite fact, as his paper included that information at the foot of the first page. Also, Norman had been requested some years after submitting his MSc to waive copyright on his thesis. He had been involved in military work during his first job after leaving university and felt he hadn't been trusted there. All these factors combined to make him suspect that there was something rather unreal and frightening about the situation. His own contribution to his thesis was minute compared to those of Carleson and others, but this didn't occur to Norman at the time.

Maybe he was overreacting to things, as he felt so elated about his own little original contributions. The fact that all his alterations had fitted so beautifully together towards the proof made him suspicious that he was meant to complete it in the way he did. He suspected that this slight variation on Carleson's proof had been known before Norman had applied himself to it. Norman believed that this version had been revealed to foreign powers after he had submitted it to the university. He thought that they might have been misled by the main original version and that the delay had been costly to them – that he had been used to lead them up the wrong path. He admired Carleson's paper on the Corona Problem so much. It was a complex and bewildering work that deserved to be remembered as having a profound application. That would show people that although this type of mathematical proof is beautiful in itself, it was not a useless effort as far as the world in general was concerned.

Norman made the decision to see his doctor. Somehow he felt that he had to convey his symptoms in a different form from how he had conveyed them to the first psychiatrist whom he had first met while at university. He decided to play down his illicit sexual entanglements, which he felt had a bearing on his present illness, and courageously discuss the medical side of his complaint. He tried to ascertain whether his type of schizophrenia was of a shift-like course as discussed in F J Fish's book on schizophrenia, but received no response from the doctor. This made him feel uncomfortable as he felt she was hiding something from him. He had interpreted Fish's view on schizophrenia as suggesting that in some cases there could be a dramatic recovery. Norman hoped that there could be an improvement in intelligence along with the recovery, and that if the psychiatrists involved with his case were right, this would be considerable – in fact, so considerable that the government would be very interested in enticing him to work for them in a military application capacity. Unfortunately he hadn't anticipated the emergence of computers, which would make the human mind practically redundant.

Despite the doctor's attempts to get him to talk about his sexual past, which he had touched on slightly, Norman refused to be drawn into supplying any details, feeling that this attitude was expected of him, as he had been too free with this type of information when he had been interrogated by the first psychiatrist he had met during the Christmas vacation when immersed in his MSc course.

The doctor was a very attractive young woman and Norman found the conversation really pleasant. After all, she was the first female he had talked intimately with for years, and hoped he had made a good impression on her. She left some of his questions unanswered but despite that the warm, friendly expression on her face, made him feel buoyant. He never had the opportunity of confiding in her again as he was transferred to another doctor in the surgery. He did notice her on a visit to his new doctor on a later date and caught her giving him a friendly glance as she passed, but no other acknowledgement.

A community psychiatric male nurse visited his flat soon afterwards. He asked Norman some further questions and details that the doctor had not covered. Sex was mentioned, and he asked Norman if he ever had any sexual relations. Norman admitted that he had had some sordid relations in the past – nothing beautiful or even pleasant. Norman asked him if any drugs existed that could result in high sexual feelings if administered and the nurse's reply was in the affirmative. This confirmed what Norman had experienced with the homosexual landlord. The nurse never returned, and Norman discovered afterwards that his 'patch' was elsewhere and that another nurse, whose area included Norman's, should have been sent as a replacement to continue Norman's treatment.

He received an appointment with the Maudsley Hospital a month later, and fortunately had by then completely recovered from his breakdown without any medical assistance being rendered to him. He still had to attend the interview and was interviewed by a junior psychiatrist. When the interview was completed, the psychiatrist summoned a consultant psychiatrist to confirm diagnosis and treatment. The latter asked Norman to show his tongue and keep it rigid for several seconds until asked to withdraw it. This was to detect tremors – a possible side effect of the medication he was taking. The consultant never gave any explanation as to why he asked Norman to stick out his tongue, and this made Norman feel uncomfortable. There was a derisory look on the consultant's face throughout and Norman felt difficult to determine what was on the latter's mind. Eventually the examination was concluded and it was with relief that Norman left the hospital. The attitude of the consultant perplexed him. Norman could only surmise that his attitude was as a result of some revelation in his records that one could find amusing. What should one expect from a person who displayed occasional bizarre symptoms due to schizophrenia? As a consultant he should have known better.

In the meantime, to Norman's horror, the bedroom ceiling started to leak. Within a matter of days the condition of the ceiling had become similar to that in which the living room ceiling had been. The water would seep in whenever it rained and the reason was the same – faulty drainage. There was no guttering, only a strip of felt over which the rainwater flowed to a vertical pipe. Apparently this system was of a bad design as the felt, through periodic exposure to the sun, was prone to develop cracks. To avoid the fusty smell of damp Norman had to remove the carpet from the bedroom floor and store it elsewhere. Thankfully he had only to wait six weeks this time before the roof was repaired. The room had been assessed by the council as unfit to live in during that period. When he replaced the carpet he discovered that it would not lie flat, but he was only relieved that the repairs had been successfully completed.

In an attempt to make his flat more pleasant to live in, Norman asked Iain to help him decorate it. They decided to start papering the bathroom with vinyl. Norman had no experience in papering a room so it was decided that Iain would take charge and teach Norman the art of decorating. It did not take Norman long to master the technique and, with Iain's supervision, he completed the decorating of the bathroom. There had been no stripping necessary as the rooms had only a coat of white distemper when he had moved in a few years previously. Within a few weeks Norman had completed the decoration of all the rooms in his flat, including the hall and kitchen, a task he relished. The transformation was spectacular and the appearance of the flat was much improved. Norman experienced a feeling of satisfaction from his efforts, and his mother admitted that she was quite pleased with the result. She expected people to redecorate every five years or so, which he did. Stripping the walls of the old paper was a very tedious chore but he enjoyed the actual papering. He partially circumvented this problem by using chip paper on the bedroom and living room walls. Then he painted over them. He was so enthusiastic about the decorating that on several occasions he would paper right through the night until he had completed the job. He simply couldn't wait to see and admire the finished product.

One morning Norman noticed a black-and-white cat on his veranda. To Norman's consternation he discovered that the cat had defecated there and this proved to be a regular occurrence. Having ascertained where the owner of the cat lived through observing the cat's movements, Norman decided to pay his neighbour a visit. His neighbour denied responsibility, claiming that there was another cat of a similar description frequenting Norman's veranda. Having made no progress from the discussion, Norman decided to report the matter to the neighbourhood office. The officer he spoke to concerning the matter suggested they erect a fence to prevent the cat from gaining access, but when Norman brought to her attention that his next door neighbour suffered the same problem, the officer seemed reluctant to include her in the arrangements. No word came from the council for some time, so Iain suggested he erect a fence himself. Some wire netting and wood staves were found and the fence was erected. To Norman's relief this appeared to deter the cat from obtaining access to Norman's veranda. When, at a later date, the council decided to renew all the drains on the estate, the fence had to be temporarily dismantled for a couple of days as scaffolding was necessary for this purpose.

The neighbour living directly beneath Norman decided to move into his partner's flat and entrusted his own flat to his partner's nephew, Peter. As soon as the nephew took over the flat he proved to be an inconsiderate neighbour. He would often invite friends into his home, and thunderous music would emanate from the flat. This would often continue into the night. To attempt to solve the problem, Norman decided to contact Environmental Health, but they did little to help. The walls used to vibrate when Peter played his deafening music. However, the original neighbour who had given over his flat to Peter was eventually evicted for running up rent arrears, and Peter was ejected from the downstairs flat. This state of affairs became evident to Norman when he noticed Peter piling his pathetic belongings into a van in order to move elsewhere. It was with a sense of relief that Norman said goodbye to him.

The crime rate was serious on the estate, and Norman was in a permanent state of anxiety about the possibility of his flat being burgled. One afternoon he heard a crashing sound from a nearby source and wondered what it was. In the evening he noticed a neighbour's door broken and off its hinges. He later discovered that that neighbour had been burgled, apparently not for the first time. The middle-aged lady living there with her family had also recently been mugged. Many other residents on the estate had been burgled during the period he remained there.

Norman's mother was so concerned about the crime rate there that she anointed the door with oil, with the symbolic sign of the cross. This cross remained on the door for years. It served as a reminder to Norman of his mother's faith, and it was certainly effective, as he was never the victim of burglary while he remained in that particular flat. He did not support his mother's Christian beliefs, but the cross on his front door made him aware of his own faults in comparison to his mother's near perfect attitude to wrongdoing. A solution to the burglary prevalent there seemed to be to take out an insurance policy on the contents of his flat, and this is what he eventually did, although the premium was quite high due to the locality.

The stairs leading up to his flat were often littered with paper foil and spent matchsticks. This indicated that drug addicts were using the relative privacy of the stairs to indulge in their craving for drugs. A street nearby was notorious for drug peddling, and it was a major problem in that area. It seemed to go on unabated. A local café was closed for its association with drugs.

'Cannabis?' asked a youth to Norman at the local bus stop.

'No thanks,' Norman politely replied, not wishing to antagonise him.

Chapter Thirteen – Change of Flat

Soon he was notified that a flat was vacant in the Stockwell area. He was quite optimistic that it would be a suitable alternative but his mother had reservations about its description. They both went to view it and he was pleased at the security of the premises, as the block had a communal entry door. The flat had also been recently refurbished. After consulting his mother he decided to accept it, but on doing so he was informed that he would not be given the option of moving back into his present estate after it was rebuilt. He had been promised that there would be a new flat available for him after the few years necessary to rebuild the estate. However, he did not argue about the situation he found himself in as he was unsatisfied with Angell Town due to its high rate of crime, and decided to give three weeks notice to the council of his intention to leave his current flat.

He made use of the intervening three weeks to have the rooms of his new flat carpeted and electricity and gas connected. He visited the flat on many mornings during the transition in order to transport fragile items by bus to his new flat and to collect any mail delivered to his new address. The windows of his new flat were half-length as compared with the full-length windows at his old address, so he made use of his mornings in the new flat to hem the old curtains to a suitable length.

At the end of the three weeks the removal company that Norman had selected came early in the morning to transport his furniture to his new abode. It was with astonishment that he watched two of them lift a heavy electric cooker into the back of the lorry, completing the task manually.

'Here is your £200 and £20 tip,' he said when the removal men had delivered the furniture to his new address.

'Thank you,' replied the foreman, accepting the money with gratitude, and adding, 'it was a pleasure. I am glad you were satisfied with our service.'

'Yes, nothing was damaged or broken in transit.'

Iain and Nora were present during most of that day and helped him to unpack. The boxes had all been marked according to their contents so that it only took a couple of hours to arrange the furniture properly. In the meantime Iain used his drill to hang up all Norman's pictures, first consulting Norman about where to place them.

Norman decided to register with a new doctor, as he was undergoing treatment with his doctor for mental health problems. There was a health clinic immediately opposite his flat and he was eventually conducted into the room of Dr Law, who was to become his new doctor.

'I always advise people in your situation that they might benefit from a review of their medical treatment. This might involve a change in medication and could involve other issues as well. I notice that you currently suffer from some side effects from the tranquilliser, pimozide, that you are on. I will arrange an appointment with a consultant psychiatrist in Saint Thomas's Hospital who will take the matter further.'

Norman thanked her and left, feeling that the future might turn out to be brighter than he had anticipated before his move. He soon received a letter detailing an appointment with Dr Davies in Saint Thomas's Hospital. As soon as Dr Davies started him on an initially minimum dose of olanzapine, problems surfaced. He was unable to get any sleep for the next few days and experienced a delusional episode, mainly centred round his previous sexual behaviour. There were some delusions regarding possible involvement by MI5 in his affairs, with Norman thinking – as before – that as Carleson's efforts on his paper on the Corona Problem had been supported by a grant from the US Airforce, there was some military application that MI5 did not want to be made public.

He continued to experience some strange symptoms during the course of the following weeks. In particular he would occasionally be attempting to complete a task when his mind would literally freeze for a few minutes, leaving his action incomplete. The symptoms caused him much distress, but it was eventually revealed to him by his psychiatrist that the behaviour he had experienced was known as 'thought withdrawal'. He had visited his general practitioner immediately this behaviour occurred but he was comforted by her reaction, which was matter of fact. She assured him that he would recover within a few weeks, and she gave the impression of having encountered these symptoms in her treatment of other patients who may have had similar medical problems. This attitude was responsible for consoling Norman and giving him hope for the future. Eventually the symptoms did subside and he was back to normality again.

During his relapses he would imagine strong disapproval from those people he made contact with from day to day. These thoughts, probably imaginary, centred round his sexual experiences in the past, which he regarded as sordid. In particular he found his guilty feelings about homosexual behaviour hard to cope with. He felt those around him knew every intimate detail of his past sexual life. He did not regard himself as a homosexual, as he felt that circumstances had brought him to the situation where he might have been tempted to indulge in such illicit sexual behaviour. His failure at finding pleasure from consorting with prostitutes had made him end up trying to find satisfaction elsewhere, but there was no pleasure in these acts for him. He also felt that the homosexual person who had deliberately slipped a drug into his drink to heighten his sexual arousal would be linked to him. He held the view that most women would find such behaviour disgusting and would reject him as a result. He was so naïve that he could not imagine what people's attitude to his sexual behaviour would be if they were to find out about it.

Dr Davies continued to experiment with the dosage of the drug he had suggested and eventually seemed to find the ideal dosage. It was essential to arrive at the minimum dosage to minimise the side effects, such as increased sugar in the blood. Norman found him very supportive, and a good listener, who gave appropriate advice as well. Most psychiatrists he had encountered previously simply asked a series of questions, noting the responses down in writing and not making any comments about them. Norman found it therapeutic to talk about his problems and was more than happy to talk regularly to medical students after his sessions with Dr Davies were over. Dr Davies would usher him in to a room to explore the techniques of interviewing with medical trainees. Norman continued his discussions with them and found that when he touched on the problem of sex their reactions were matter of fact. He would depart with mixed feelings. On the one hand he would derive comfort from the fact that they had reacted so calmly to his revelations, on the other he felt disturbed at bringing up these experiences from the past.

On the whole he felt regret and repentance with his past sexual behaviour, and there was relevance with the first painting that one encounters on one's way into the National Gallery. This is a painting by Gian Savoldo of Saint Jerome inflicting blows on his chest to ward off evil thoughts. It was comforting in a sense to realise that even a saint could have wrong thoughts. If Norman had been able to dispel his thoughts about his past sexual life from his mind he would have resorted to anything to give himself peace of mind.

In the picture, Saint Jerome kneels in front of a crucifix, seemingly asserting that our path through life should be the narrow one, focusing on Jesus for salvation. Everything else comes a poor second. The painting alongside it is by the same painter and again it has a religious theme. The painting shows Mary Magdalene at the tomb where Jesus was buried. She is illuminated by a light emanating from a supernatural source, possibly indicating the presence of Jesus. She seems to shrink from his appearance. Her intention was to anoint his body but the realisation comes eventually that he is risen... We should serve Jesus as we can during our brief lives here on earth, and those who trust him can rest assured of his forgiveness after repentance of our past sins.

In the meantime, after settling into his new flat for several months Norman heard a knock one day on his door. It was his next door neighbour, Lucy, introducing herself. She was an elderly lady in her nineties. Eventually Norman became aware of carers visiting her and quite often they would ring his buzzer to gain access to her, as Lucy was profoundly deaf and had difficulty communicating. They would do her shopping regularly, based on a shopping list she would make. It transpired that she had cats which she doted on. She made the comment later that unlike humans cats don't answer back or deliberately hurt one's feelings. It was touching to see how attached she was to her cats; they seemed to be the only companions and friends she had. Their welfare seemed to be foremost in her mind, as she always made sure that she included adequate food supplies for them when composing her shopping lists. It transpired later that she suffered from senile dementia.

A carer from Nigeria called Comfort, who visited Lucy regularly, became the first person for many years to make a relationship with Norman that was not merely just superficial. Sometimes Comfort would seek advice from Norman about the shopping lists Lucy provided her, Lucy's writing being difficult to read. Comfort was unfamiliar with English and found communication a major problem. She confided in Norman that she was a Christian and urged Norman to start going to church. He rejected her advice. Her name seemed strangely appropriate as she really was a source of comfort to all around her, including Norman. On her visits to Lucy she would call on Norman's flat and spend some time in conversation with him. She had the endearing habit of looking into his fridge and requesting a packet of biscuits or a bottle of Coke to take away with her. Norman was quite happy to comply with her requests. It made him feel closer to her; she was willing to accept something he could provide. Her motives, in practically seizing these items of food, may have been deliberately designed to make Norman feel he had something she wanted, perhaps his friendship only.

One morning Norman noticed a few itchy lumps on his legs. The sensation was unbearable and he could not resist scratching them. More lumps appeared over a period of several weeks, and he was puzzled about their origin, assuming he had developed an allergic reaction to some food. However, to his horror, one day he noticed a small black flea on his leg. The flea jumped off when Norman attempted to catch it and examine it. It dawned on him that he had involuntarily carried some cat fleas on his person from Lucy's flat, and that they had subsequently bred in his flat. This was confirmed when another neighbour called Stephen confided that he was plagued with the same problem.

'No matter how desperate her need is,' Stephen asserted, 'I will never enter her premises again.'

'I do not feel I can abandon her at this stage,' Norman replied. 'She still depends on me to assist her with her shopping. I will contact the Pest Control Department and get them to eradicate the creatures from our premises.'

There ensued a long wait of three weeks before the pest control officer came and fumigated all the flats in the block. The problem continued, and he had to be summoned back a second time in order to treat the premises again.

His problems with his neighbour Lucy did not end there. Despite all his efforts to help her she persisted in communicating with him via notes pushed through his letter box, in which she accused him, among many other things, of being a whoremonger. That description was unconfirmed as she knew nothing about Norman's past. She also accused him in her letters of having 'a factory' on his premises that caused excessive noise. She was profoundly deaf, so it appeared that her deafness caused her to experience noise in her ears. Her behaviour was symptomatic of dementia.

One day she wrote down a sexual suggestion in one of her notes. After giving the matter considerable thought he decided to respond positively to her request for sex. He wrote an encouraging reply on the other side of her note and pushed it through her door. This turned out to be futile, as the only response he had from her was a note threatening to inform the council about his own response. This was rather worrying for him as he dreaded having the situation made public, making him appear a fool. He had only responded to her as she had apparently hoped for, and her reaction was obviously linked with her dementia.

He decided not to enter her flat again, as her cats had not received flea treatment, and the danger of re-infestation remained. After shunning her flat for a week she came to Norman's door and Norman decided not to answer.

'Norman, please…' she announced brokenly, and then returned to her flat. The incident was so harrowing for him that he was reduced to tears when relating the event to his mother next day. Several days afterwards Lucy was visited by a doctor, as she had been confined to bed and was unable to get up. The doctor came to Norman's door and said that if Lucy did not cooperate and agree to be transferred to the local hospital for treatment, she would die within a few weeks. Apparently she had refused hospital treatment.

A psychiatrist soon came to visit her to ascertain whether she was of sound mind to make her own decision regarding hospital treatment. She was assessed as being capable of making the decision for herself and so she remained in her flat.

Three weeks later Norman attended her funeral. She had no living relatives, and those who attended her funeral were neighbours only. Norman was sad in a sense that she had died but felt a sense of relief that her behaviour towards him, which caused so much distress, was finally over. The day of the funeral was quite a pleasant day and the cloud formation in the sky reminded him of the depiction in the sky in the well known painting by Vermeer called 'A View of Delft'. The same feeling of quiet and stillness depicted in the painting, and which the reflection of the buildings in the canal evoked, was present during the funeral service. Sadly she could not claim –

> Where is death's sting? Where, grave, thy victory?
> I triumph still if Thou abide with me.

The hymn summed up the sadness of the event. She was referred to, by those who knew her, as a lapsed Catholic.

Chapter Fourteen – Attempt at Rehabilitation

When Norman expressed a desire to Dr Davies to attempt employment again, he suggested Norman attend the Mosaic Clubhouse – a rehabilitation centre focusing on helping its members return to work. Dr Davies made contact with them on Norman's behalf and Norman received a letter from the Clubhouse after a few weeks had elapsed.

On arrival at the centre, he was ushered into a room where several others had arrived with the intention of becoming members themselves. The object of the first visit was to be shown round the centre by an established member. Those who had arrived with Norman for that purpose had to make a decision whether to become members or not. It transpired that the centre was involved in running about twenty jobs through external contacts with employers. They were known as 'transitional employments', as the object was to introduce members to supported work and then encourage them to seek independent employment. The jobs, only a few of which were unfilled at any given time, carried a basic wage and were part-time.

The centre had a café and provided meals and refreshments at a subsidised price. The running of the Clubhouse was through active participation of members alongside a staff of about six. This gave those members involved in the running of the centre experience in relating to people in a type of work environment. Norman was introduced to a computer and was shown how to use spreadsheets to record the daily attendance of the members. On an average day there would be about thirty members attending. Norman was advised that a twice-weekly attendance at least was advisable, so he attended the centre twice a week.

It was not easy at the beginning to relate to the other members, as they suffered from mental health problems themselves, and were similar to Norman in finding it difficult to make relationships with other people. However they all coexisted amicably and he found some that he could become on friendly terms with. In particular there he met a lady called Eileen, with whom he got on with quite well. She would accompany him on the journey back home, as she lived only a few blocks away from him. She had a nice sense of humour that he found appealing. Sometimes she would visit him in his flat but it was just a platonic relationship. She was about sixty and there was no strong physical attraction there between them. She was quite a good conversationalist and he felt comfortable with someone like that. He always made a point of finding something relevant in response to her chatter and this encouraged her to continue. She had been diagnosed as having schizophrenia like him. He felt an empathy with all the members as he had experienced the problems of mental illness himself and knew how much suffering could be involved.

He also encountered a female at the rehabilitation centre called Dawn. She happened to be the first female he had ever gone out on a date with. She herself suggested a visit to the local pub, to which Norman agreed. She had to have the support of a stick, as her walking had been affected by a previous accident, from which she had not yet recovered. They went to the cinema and paid several visits to a pub. Norman felt resentful because she never offered to pay towards the cost of the entertainment; he also found her to be quite unattractive. She would often ask him for a loan, but to her credit, she always repaid it. On one occasion she threatened to go begging if she did not receive the loan asked for. Norman refused on this occasion. There was also a disagreement between them as to whether one loan had been paid in full. Their paths diverged and the words of Polonius came to his mind:

> Neither a borrower nor a lender be;
> For loan oft loses both itself and friend.

He familiarised himself with the very basics of computers at the centre. The centre possessed several that were used by members for various tasks. Iain happened to be upgrading own computer at that time and offered him the old computer that he was replacing. Norman accepted and Iain installed it for him. He found a website on the computer that sold art reproductions and decided to buy some, to be delivered through the post. He could see a preview on the computer screen. The most appealing reproductions were by Renoir and Monet. His favourite was 'Two Sisters' by Renoir, which he bought and had framed.

He developed an interest in the history of art and decided to attend classes on art at Putney College one evening a week. He made copious notes but found it difficult to retain factual information in his mind. He found dates very difficult to memorise. The classes covered the emergence of American art over the recent centuries. He found the majority of those who attended the classes were middle class and difficult to relate to. There was a break for refreshments in the college café at the halfway point of the lecture.

'I wonder why the vast majority of artists who have been successful artists have usually been composed of men,' he uttered impulsively to one lady in the class as they were all queuing up for tea.

'That is simply not true,' she retorted brusquely, and continued in an unpleasant tone, 'what about Berthe Morisot and Georgia O'Keeffe?'

Norman felt hurt by her tone of voice and felt more of an outsider than before. However, his confidence in his ability to take notes improved, in contrast to his past difficulties as a pupil at school and university. He had never visited an art gallery during his nine months' course on art, but vowed he would eventually go. The computer he had received had been instrumental in his budding interest in the history of art.

He made a decision about that time to learn how to play bridge. He had attempted briefly to learn it thirty years ago but had failed to understand the logic behind the bidding. He felt that if he applied himself diligently to learn it he would be successful. He managed to download a bridge playing program on his computer and was delighted at his apparent skill at playing. He could not completely understand the bidding so he made the decision to join a bridge club and take it from there. After some inquiries on the Internet he opted for the Andrew Robson Bridge Club and, one evening, during a visit from his mother, he decided to visit the club for an introductory session for beginners intending to make a decision to take up bridge seriously.

He was positioned at a table with some staff members who felt his bidding needed considerable improvement. After several games they left the table and he was left alone on the periphery of those present. He remained there for about an hour, feeling as if he had been excluded, until he finally decided to leave. When he arrived back at his flat he revealed his disappointment to his mother; he felt he had been rejected by the bridge club for some unknown reason. Next day he suffered from a relapse and had to seek medical help. His psychiatrist told him that his experience in the bridge club was not necessarily the cause of his breakdown. Apparently other factors played their parts.

He persevered at the bridge club and decided to take lessons there. The lessons cost about £150 for a series of eight, and he decided to tackle the intermediate course first. He continued and made good progress until he reached the final and most advanced course, after which he brushed up his conventions at £20 a session. He never regretted his outlay in learning bridge, as his knowledge of the game enabled him to derive enormous pleasure from it into the future.

Meanwhile it had been suggested to him at the rehabilitation centre that he should start a therapeutic employment job. He complied with the suggestion and he started paid part-time work for an organisation that provided videos for potential investors on the stock exchange. The work was very elementary and simply consisted of erasing videotapes. The job had been clearly explained to him by a member of the Mosaic Clubhouse called Janet. It was a start, and he would possibly have floundered in any other demanding job at that time. He had an embarrassing encounter there with an Asian girl called Pritti when he had occasion to ask her, 'Are you Pritti?' He made no friendships there, possibly because his work did not involve other people.

After working in that capacity for six months, he was allocated by the centre work for a health authority. The job was run by the centre, which was responsible for the training involved. The work involved printing medical information using several large printers, and some computer work involving medical records of patients under that health authority. The printers had to be linked up in a preparatory fashion to the computers before the printing process and that was quite involved. Anne, another member of the Mosaic Clubhouse, didn't explain the procedure as Norman would have liked it to be explained, but he persevered and finally mastered it.

At the health authority he met another member of Mosaic called Sabina. She had the same illness as him, having suffered for a considerable time with schizophrenia. She took the same medication. It was Norman's task to explain the work to her but she found it difficult to grasp. Norman made an extra effort to assist her, as he had encountered learning problems during previous employments himself. At times he would stay behind for an extra hour or so to acquaint her with what was required. By the time he had left the job she had managed to grasp the essentials of it. She was such a sweet natured person, and Norman liked her enormously. Unfortunately she was thirty years younger than Norman and so a closer relationship seemed out of the question to him. She had a passion for chocolate and professed a liking for the dark kind. She asserted that she was a Christian and once asked Norman out of the blue, 'Do you know Crefflo Dollar?'

'Yes,' Norman replied, continuing, 'I have come across that evangelist through my mother's viewing of Christian channels.'

He found her conversation sweet and endearing. There were several other Christians among the permanent staff, and one called Dionne was kind enough to present him with a card and a box of chocolates when he left that organisation. He respected those Christians as they somehow reminded him of his mother, who happened to be a Christian herself. The supervisor, Rose, was very cooperative and was always happy to answer any question that might arise regarding the work. He felt an affinity with the Christians there, as they stood out as being better in their outlook and behaviour generally. Although he was beginning to feel that his life was about to improve, he immediately should have heeded, from that point on until he became a Christian, the comment made regarding the man who decided to tear down his barns and build new ones to make room for his good harvest, thinking he would eat, drink and be merry for many years to come.

'You fool! This very night your life will be demanded from you. Then who will get what you have prepared for yourself?'

Having gained some confidence through his experiences doing therapeutic employment, Norman decided to investigate the possibility of independent employment. As a result of some enquiries, an employment agency known as Status Employment was recommended to him. They specialised in finding employment for people with mental health issues. Their staff was very friendly and helpful. They suggested visiting the employment exchange and introduced Norman to the Disablement Replacement Officer. On one visit a member of Status accompanied him during an interview with an employment exchange staff member called Milly.

'What type of work would interest you?' she asked, after Norman had furnished her with some details regarding his educational qualifications and work experience.

'I do not want to attempt anything too stressful. The process of learning the job seems to have been a problem for me in the past. I want to learn from my previous mistakes, so to err on the side of caution I will opt for a job as a filing clerk. I feel confident I can cope with that kind of work as I do not envisage learning it to be a problem.'

'Are you certain in your own mind that you would not get bored with such work? You do have some high educational qualifications, Norman.'

'In the past I found supervisors unapproachable, and filing requires the minimum of instruction.'

After checking on the available work on offer, the employment officer came up with a part-time job as a filing clerk in a doctor's surgery. Norman accepted this opportunity, and an appointment for an interview was made for him over the phone for the following day.

Next day Norman donned his best suit and arrived at the surgery twenty minutes early. Eventually the practice manager, Helen, ushered him into a room, where she and a surgery doctor called Dr Hope began his interview. Helen seemed to him uncertain about his suitability, but Norman sensed that Dr Hope was influenced by various factors in regarding him as suitable.

Norman confessed during the interview that he had had mental health problems during the past. Dr Hope asked him what medication he was taking, and Norman admitted that he took olanzapine. The practice manager might not have been aware of what illness the drug was prescribed for, but obviously Dr Hope knew. He was told he would be contacted the next day, and indeed, next day he received a letter offering him the job.

Norman was delighted at this and immediately wrote a letter of acceptance. On arrival on his first day at work he was introduced to the rest of the staff. His work consisted of filing the documents that were received by the surgery on a daily basis, from hospitals that treated patients who belonged to that particular surgery. The documents had to be filed and deposited into filing cabinets in alphabetical order according to the patient's surname. There was also a considerable amount of test results to be filed as well.

Jennifer, who worked for the surgery on a computer, was quite friendly. She was kind enough to assist him on his first day with the filing. He worked on his feet daily for 3½ hours, and at first the continual bending to reach the cabinets at floor level caused him to feel dizzy. This feeling persisted for several weeks but eventually faded away. The area in which he worked was situated behind the reception area. There was an array of filing cabinets arranged in a square into which all documents were placed. Initially there was a backlog but he managed to eliminate this and was eventually more or less up to date. There was sufficient work coming in on a daily basis to keep him occupied. He had been informed that a previous filing clerk had been unable to cope with the volume of documents coming into the surgery, and that even the surgery doctors had had to lend a hand to get the filing under control. It had taken them several weeks to get up to date. Norman was pleased that he was able to cope with the amount of documents which were coming in regularly every day.

As far as the members of staff there was concerned he seemed to have an adequate relationship with them. However, he felt uncomfortable with one female called Pauline. She would occasionally exhibit the unpleasant habit of interrupting his conversation with other people, and sometimes walk off when he was addressing her. Norman's counsellor asked him to consider the possibility that she might dislike him. This was something Norman found difficult to accept as he had never entertained that possibility about anyone. On exploring what motives Pauline might have had for disliking him the counsellor suggested that he might have reminded Pauline of someone from her past whom presumably she had abhorred. This seemed to Norman to be a feeble explanation for the situation that existed between Pauline and himself.

It transpired that two of the doctors there were gay, along with two of the male receptionists. One of these receptionists, called Luigi, was very popular with the female members of staff. Norman found that their encouragement of Luigi's lifestyle was a bit hard to swallow. They would discuss his current boyfriends with him as if this was an ordinary and accepted type of conversation. The fact that they condoned and encouraged Luigi's homosexuality made Norman feel that there was little opportunity for him to create enduring relationships with the opposite sex. He felt some women appeared to prefer homosexuals to heterosexuals. He had read that women feel less threatened by gay men and often established friendships with them. He felt many women preferred gay men and yet would reject any man who was not completely heterosexual. He overheard Helen say on one occasion, 'You make your bed and you lie in it,' and felt this might be directed at him. On another occasion he heard her refer to someone as a schizophrenic in scathing terms. This could have been a patient, but Norman still felt affronted.

Soon after starting his part-time work, Norman was invited to the Clubhouse to give a speech on his experiences at finding and coping with independent work. He prepared a speech, which he read out during an employment dinner there. Those members who were present applauded him afterwards and he hoped he had been instrumental in encouraging them to make an effort to find work themselves. He knew that for those who suffered from mental health problems the inability to hold down a permanent job was an ever present problem for them. It made them feel more isolated in the community. Following Norman, another member delivered a speech on his own experiences. He had not prepared his speech but Norman congratulated him on his courage, as a previous teacher of history, in continuing in that area after experiencing mental health problems.

Chapter Fifteen – Entertainment

Norman decided to spend a considerable amount of the money he was earning on entertainment, especially theatre visits. He also accumulated a considerable sum towards his savings to prepare him for the inevitable event of retirement. He was fortunate enough to qualify for tax credit and this benefit boosted his income considerably. He would visit the theatres alone, having come to a decision about what to see through theatre information on the Internet. He felt it a challenge to mix and go places. This was different from his attitude in previous years. He felt the urge to persevere in his relationships, although at times some of his dealings with people proved difficult. He seemed to be getting benefits from his associations, though some were intricate and more difficult to develop in his point of view.

Once he watched a musical called *Bombay Dreams* and was attracted by the couple of Indian-type songs that were performed. On returning home he made enquiries through the internet regarding the purchase of Bollywood DVDs. Each Bollywood DVD treated sex discreetly, and the simplicity of their approach to sex attracted him. He appreciated the Asian music and found the songs catchy. His favourite was *Hamara Dil Aapke Paas Hai* featuring Aishwarya Rai and Anil Kapoor. This particular movie portrayed a very romantic encounter between the two as the title song was played. Their friendship was so beautiful and their obvious attraction for each other was intensified by the haunting music. All the Bollywood films he bought had English subtitles.

His interest in music became extended to opera. He somehow felt that by extending and increasing his general interests he would find more in common with those people he associated with and make conversation flow easier. His favourite opera was *The Merry Widow*, which he played often. The musical talent of the composer impressed him, as practically all the arias were beautiful and original. He enjoyed light operas like Gilbert and

Sullivan and visited some performances of their operas in various theatres including *The Pirates of Penzance* and *The Mikado*. He loved the humour of the libretti and bought a compilation of all their libretti in a massive book. The humour became more apparent through reading the volume.

Eventually he made a decision to visit The National Gallery – his first visit to an art gallery. He was pleasantly surprised at what was on offer, and tended to find the Christian art especially appealing and moving. He was surprised at the vast collection of books on art in the gallery's three bookshops and was to buy many books from that source. The books he purchased covered all the main artists throughout the centuries back to about the time of Cimabue. He was delighted to discover that free guided tours were on offer twice a day; he preferred these rather than going round the gallery on his own. The tour guides gave an intelligent commentary on about five paintings and he found their style of English very attractive. Their commentaries brought the paintings to life. Even still life paintings like those on view by Menendez would come to life under the scrutiny of the tour guides.

He would have a break halfway through his visit and enjoy a pot of tea and cake in the gallery café. The restaurant was very expensive as far as he was concerned, but he did have a few meals there on occasions when he had more money than usual to spend. The ribeye steak he settled for was beautifully prepared and cooked, and despite the price he felt happy at the quality of the meal. It was something he would like to indulge in only occasionally. He extended his interest in art by visiting other art galleries in London, but found that The National Gallery was preferable, as audio guides were available at a cheap price and covered practically all the paintings on view.

After spending a year filing he was told that the system was to change and that the documents would be scanned into the patients' records on a computer in the future. A female from the Health Authority took the opportunity for two hours to instruct Norman, Jennifer and Helen to scan the documents and enter their details on the computer under the corresponding patient.

After scanning, the documents were to be deposited in boxes in the typist's room. The typist was a Jehovah's Witness. She seemed to disapprove of the system of disposing of the documents and suggested to Norman storing the documents in a large cabinet. Norman did not want to disagree with her and felt like saying he was just carrying out the practice manager's instructions. Instead he made no comment on the situation. He hated openly disagreeing with people as this could easily develop into a heated argument, a situation he avoided at all costs. He felt if this occurred he would end up on the losing side.

The other gay receptionist, Dan, was, unlike Luigi, rather unpopular in the surgery. One day Norman approached him, knowing that he was gay, and asked him if he found women physically attractive. Dan replied that he only reacted to women who were particularly beautiful and distinctive, such as film stars. Norman regarded himself as being at the heterosexual end of the sex scale, for as a rule he only found women physically attractive. Norman would occasionally be drawn to men who would be extremely handsome, but he put this down to a feeling of jealousy on his part. Sometimes it was difficult for him to assess and understand his own feelings. Dan didn't seem to take offence at Norman's question and Norman was struck by his politeness. Norman felt uncomfortable as he liked both Dan and Luigi as people in themselves. They both seemed to have nice personalities. No wonder the female staff found them appealing! He was to repeat the same question to Luigi a year later, but unfortunately Luigi seemed to take offence at this and his attitude to Norman cooled somewhat. Maybe Luigi felt Norman was critical of his sexual orientation.

Helen suggested to Norman that he might assist a member of the staff, Val, to complete the tagging of documents. This involved going through all the files in the surgery, putting the documents in each patient's file in date order, after putting them also into various categories. They would then be forwarded to a Dr Louis, who would be responsible for summarising the contents of each patient's records on the computer. Val had already tagged the majority of the files and Norman was asked to deal with the tagging of the new patients' files, while Val proceeded with the previously established patients' records. Norman and Val shared an upstairs room for five hours every Monday, when Norman dealt with the new patient files for that week. The rest of the week he was solely involved in scanning documents.

Val confided in him that she was living with a partner called Chris. She was on friendly terms with one of the gay doctors called Dave. Norman found Dave a likeable person as well, and Dave would always greet Norman with a warm smile. This made Norman feel slightly uncomfortable but at the same time flattered. Norman was forced to examine his own sexual position and hoped that his liking for Dave had no sexual overtones. The fact that Norman found it easier to make relationships with males rather than females caused him some concern. Women could be on the defensive when interacting with males... Val herself was in her mid-seventies and her partner was ten years younger. She was kind enough to invite Norman to her home and take him to a local restaurant where they both, with Chris in tow, had a meal. Norman returned the favour by inviting both of them to his flat, after which he took the couple to a local Indian restaurant. Val and Chris seemed to be a very happy couple and Norman had to admit to feeling a trifle jealous as he observed them making eye contact with each other and smiling pleasurably at one another over the meals. Norman enjoyed the evening but felt he had stood out as he had no female companion to make up a foursome. It made him more acutely aware that he had no close relationships with a female whom he could have invited along.

Dr Louis, the doctor who was responsible for the summarising, was a qualified doctor from Sri Lanka. He had been unable to find work as a doctor in this country. Norman had quite a friendly relationship with him and Louis expressed an interest in learning how to play bridge. Norman agreed to spend some time coaching him, but Louis' efforts proved to be of no avail and he decided to abandon his attempt. It may have been that Norman could not convey his bridge knowledge satisfactorily to Louis. Louis knew of Norman's admiration for Asian women, and offered to find Norman an Asian wife.

'I think I could look into the possibility of finding you an

Asian lady who would be very happy about a marriage arrange-ment. I have contacts and am certain that there are many out there who would jump at the chance of an arranged marriage.'

Norman declined Louis' offer, as he felt unable to support a female on his limited income. In any case Norman had spent most of his life living a solitary lifestyle and would find it difficult to share his life with another. The suggestion had its attractive side as Norman had had never had a sexual outlet, and had in fact not had any sexual encounters for over forty years. However, he felt people on the whole might regard him as being sexually active, not knowing the truth. In any case he had become a Christian, and as a result he believed sex was only acceptable within a marriage.

Chapter Sixteen – Bridge for Fun

The first couple of years playing in the bridge club were difficult ones for Norman. He had not attended the beginners' course, having felt that he had enough knowledge of the game to start with the intermediate course. The etiquette involved in the mixing, cutting and dealing of the two packs of cards allocated to each table were covered only in the beginners' course. As a result Norman was unable to grasp this effectively, being unable even to understand it from continued practice. He always felt embarrassed before every game, as he had to rely on the others to enlighten him as far as this preliminary stage of the game was concerned. Eventually he decided to join the more advanced sessions and play duplicate bridge. There, the hands were already prepared, and each player received a set hand which was repeated at other tables. No dealing was required.

One morning during a lesson at the bridge club on bridge conventions a portly and bearded man introduced himself to Norman as Eddie. He said that his bridge tutor, Simon, had suggested he play on a regular basis with Norman as Simon felt both their styles were compatible. He revealed that his wife was Susan Hampshire, the actress. Eddie and Norman were to play together most Thursday mornings for many years. Norman found Eddie to be a polite and distinguished man and soon found out that Eddie was probably the most liked and popular member of the bridge club. It transpired at a later time that Eddie was in fact a knight, having been knighted by Prince Charles, possibly for Eddie's generous support to athletics and the arts. He had lavished literally millions of pounds on these causes. It was a very happy and productive partnership, and Norman had many happy occasions playing with Eddie. Once Eddie noticed Norman buying a brand of chocolate at the bridge club and showed his kindness by buying one every Thursday morning, when they would both share it at a convenient lull in the bridge session.

Eventually, after some years, he discontinued producing it out of his shirt pocket, outwardly because he had decided that it would be undesirable as he was overweight, but inwardly possibly because he felt he might be regarded as a trifle childish in regularly buying that particular brand of chocolate. Eddie's attitude to money was a sensible one, despite the fact that he was a millionaire. Norman had confided in Eddie that he did not envy rich people and that he was content with a low income.

'A man's life does not consist in the abundance of his possessions.'

On one occasion Eddie kindly invited Norman with many others from the bridge club to watch a performance of his wife on stage. Norman had been seated next to a lady called Serena, whom he had met at the bridge club previously. He had made the observation to her, after she had revealed that her alias on Internet bridge was Mona Lisa, that he might have known that fact from her intriguing smile. She had responded to his remark favourably. However after the intermission she walked off and engaged someone else in conversation. Norman felt she had snubbed him but did not let that cause him any sorrow or pain as he was relieved that the responsibility of making conversation with her was lifted. The words of Hamlet to Polonius when the latter expressed a wish to take his leave of Hamlet came to his mind.

> You cannot, sir [or madam, as the case may have been], take from me anything that I will not more willingly part withal – except my life, except my life, except my life.

After the show Eddie drove Norman to a restaurant that had been booked for the occasion. He had invited about twenty-five people there. Norman sat next to Averil, who was another member of the bridge club. During the meal Norman was unable to make conversation with the lady sitting opposite him and Averil remarked that Norman was one of Eddie's favourites and that 'still waters ran deep'. At a later date Norman would remind Averil of this incident and say that he hoped that one day he would be regarded as 'a bubbling brook in the springtime', a comparison he had encountered on reading a book on psycho-somatic medicine called *The Person in the Body*.

For a couple of years previous to this incident, Norman had been accompanying his half-brother Iain and mother Nora to their local church on Sundays. They had finally succeeded in persuading him to join them there regularly. The services moved him and on occasions the readings referring to Jesus' suffering caused tears to well up in his eyes. The preachers revealed the beauty of the Scriptures through their discussion and analysis of them. In particular the many metaphors involving water made an impact on him. It made him realise that the Scriptures could match and surpass any book by the most accomplished writer. Even Shakespeare paled into insignificance in comparison to the Bible. He did feel uncomfortable near the end of the service, because he was unable to come forward for communion as he was technically an unbeliever. A dear elderly lady called Ellen, who would shake hands with the each member of the congregation as they exited through the door of the church, made an impression on him. She would clasp his hands warmly and utter kind words to him. No one else responded to him like she did. Her attitude influenced his decision at a later time to become a Christian. He would be reminded of a telling few lines of Scripture from Luke, that were spoken by Jesus and are as follows: 'I praise you father, Lord of heaven and earth, because you have hidden these things from the wise and learned, and revealed them to little children. Yes, Father, for this was your good pleasure.'

In the meantime, Iain, having just moved into that area due to experiencing excessive noise and disturbance in their previous flat, decided to get in touch with a lady called Pauline, who lived in Manchester. He met her through a Christian dating agency. He had bought a house in East Ham, not outright, having to pay a mortgage on it. It was within his financial ability to cope with the mortgage as he had saved enough from his employment to put down a considerable deposit on it. He was receiving an ample salary at that time through his work as a computer specialist.

Iain showed Norman Pauline's picture on the Internet site. She looked very beautiful with lovely long dark hair. After Iain had visited her in Manchester several times they decided to get engaged. They decided to marry but the marriage had to be postponed due to the sudden death of Pauline's father. After a subsequent lapse of time, the marriage was rescheduled and Norman was asked to be best man at the wedding. Iain and Norman visited a tailor who measured them for wedding suits which were for hire. They even had matching blue ties, a colour Pauline had chosen.

Norman prepared his short wedding speech beforehand and was considerably helped by Iain, who made some suggestions regarding the content of the speech. The wedding went smoothly and at the reception Norman successfully delivered his speech. There was prolonged applause afterwards. He was sitting during the wedding banquet next to Iain on his left, and Doreen – Pauline's aunt – on his right. It was later disclosed to Norman that Doreen suffered from depression, having recently lost her husband. She seemed happy and talkative at the wedding, but within a matter of months her condition deteriorated and she was permanently admitted to a nursing home. Her decline in health was tragic and extremely painful for her immediate family.

Iain moved up to a rural area in Macclesfield, Cheshire, where he was able to buy a house outright. It was situated twenty miles south of Manchester, where Pauline lived. Pauline continued residing with her mother who had not fully recovered from her husband's death. Pauline was very supportive and encouraging to Norman, never criticising his fondness for bridge, and kept praying that his interest in bridge would develop successfully. His mother, on the other hand, found it difficult to give her approval, as she probably associated card games with gambling and this ran counter to her Christian faith.

Chapter Seventeen – Christianity

When Iain moved to Macclesfield, Norman decided to continue his churchgoing on his own. He decided to visit church regularly and ventured to attend a local Baptist church one Sunday. However, the congregation was practically all black and he did not receive a warm welcome there. The main reason he had for not returning was that the preacher there regarded the display of crosses in church as idolatry. This view seemed to Norman to be very extreme and he felt he would not be comfortable there.

The following Sunday he visited a church that was Church of England, called Saint Anne and All Saints. The congregation there was mixed and he received a warmer welcome there. The vicar, Ailsa, talked to him briefly as he left the church. She suggested a regular discussion group at her vicarage to explore his budding Christian faith. There, Norman and another two aspiring Christians, Bill and Jim, would meet to discuss Christian issues, and prepare for eventual confirmation. Norman found the discussions helpful, and Ailsa was able to address some doubts he had. He felt he was making the right decision to approach confirmation in this way; he also felt that confirmation would bring home to him the necessity of making a definite commitment to trust in Jesus as his personal saviour. Bill and Norman decided to be confirmed at Southwark Cathedral at Easter but Jim did not. Jim's views seemed nebulous and his points of view on Christian matters seemed illogical. His arguments did not reach for a clear conclusion and his train of thought was difficult to follow.

Norman felt so influenced by the sermons and Christian attitude in general that he decided to visit a bookshop – the CLC – to search for a CD which would include the hymn 'God is Love'. The verses of the hymn seemed to speak to him personally and the tune was so attractive. Sadly, the bookshop assistants were unable to find the hymn in their stock. In his search for God the second verse seemed to have resonance for him:

None can see God above;
Neighbours here we can love;
Thus may we Godward move,
Finding him in others,
Sisters all, and brothers.

He was to return to that bookshop several months later and divulge to the staff there that he was now a Christian. They revealed that they had prayed for him after his first visit there, that he might find Jesus.

On Easter day, Norman and Bill were confirmed, along with many others, by Bishop Tom at Southwark Cathedral. As Norman knelt down, and Bishop Tom placed his hand on Norman's head to confirm him, Norman felt the power of the Holy Spirit enter him. After the confirmation, Ailsa, who was present, kindly provided the three with their certificates of confirmation and Christian books commemorating the occasion.

The congregation at Saint Anne's were quite welcoming and before very long Norman felt relaxed and happy with his visits there. Ailsa introduced him to a lady in the congregation named Irene. Irene coincidentally came from Stornoway, the capital of the Isle of Lewis. This town was only seven miles distant from the village Norman was brought up in. They exchanged experiences they had encountered at school, it having transpired that they had both attended the same school. She revealed that she often visited her relatives back there, and was surprised when Norman revealed that he had never returned there since the time he had left forty-five years ago.

Norman began his involvement with the affairs of the church at an early point of his attendance there. He was very happy to volunteer to do the church cleaning there once a month. A rota was established and he found himself doing the cleaning with different people from time to time, two people sharing the task. The humility required to perform this task somehow appealed to him. Unfortunately, one lady who was supposed to assist him failed to turn up on several occasions without contacting him in advance to give an explanation of why she couldn't come. On these occasions he had to do the cleaning alone. He found it rather tiring but felt a strange feeling of joy and pleasure that he was doing something constructive for the church. Due to the failure of volunteers to be present when they should have been, it was eventually decided to employ and pay a lady to do it on a weekly basis. Norman was congratulated by Michael, a church-warden, on his perfect attendance in his task of doing the cleaning, as compared to others who were not so reliable.

As Norman continued to grow as a Christian he would often visit the CLC for Christian material. This would consist of reading material, videos or DVDs. He was to develop a thirst for exploring the bible through commentaries. He amassed quite a collection of Christian books and also many books on artists and the history of art. Most paintings in the fourteenth to sixteenth centuries seemed to revolve around Christianity and there was a very good selection of that type of art in the National Gallery.

Ailsa suggested to Norman that he might like to be responsible for writing the weekly cheques for the church expenses, and fill in the associated forms. He was eager to do this. Soon afterwards, Ailsa asked him if he would like to take charge of the church accounts. Norman assented to this and in due course was visited by Charlie, who had done them in the past. Charlie attempted to introduce Norman to the method of doing the accounts and spent about an hour discussing it, using Norman's computer, on which he had set the accounts up. Charlie laboured over the same points and in the end had achieved very little. Several months passed during which Norman had no further visits from Charlie. It was decided that David, the person currently doing the accounts, should visit Norman and show how to enter the accounts on computer. David came several times and Norman was gradually able to take over the accounts. Norman confided in David that he thought Charlie did not appear to have much confidence in Norman's ability to do the work.

One Sunday morning, which seemed like any other, Norman entered the church and sat down in his usual place in a pew. After a few minutes the thought came into his mind that on his entrance to the church he had seen Ailsa at the back of the church smoking a cigarette held in a cigarette holder. The thought seemed so real that he could visualise in his mind the smoke curling up into the atmosphere from her cigarette. The experience upset him enormously, as he feared he might be experiencing regular hallucinations and that he might not be able to distinguish fact from fantasy. He was uncertain as to whether the experience had had been indicative of memory impairment, or whether he had actually had a hallucination. He confided in Bill, as he was desperate for advice, and also approached Ailsa herself about the matter, revealing what had happened to him. She stated that she did not smoke. Norman feared he could not depend on his senses and that this type of incident might keep recurring. He dreaded how his mind could develop and that possibly the boundary between reality and unreality might not be a distinct one. Fortunately, nothing similar happened subsequently, although the memory of the event remained with him permanently.

Some months afterwards when the accounts had been entrusted to Norman, the church decided to award David a season ticket for the Royal Academy, and his wife a bouquet of flowers, for their efforts. Norman was able to take over successfully but initially had to clarify some points, which he wrote down and presented to Ailsa. He was disappointed and upset by her reaction. She brusquely stated that these matters were not within her sphere now, and that any questions should be directed at Sasha, a church member who was involved in church finances. He found it more difficult to approach her than he had been accustomed to, but apart from that incident he found her a hard working and caring vicar. Again he might have read more into that incident than it warranted and felt he should have understood the pressure Ailsa was under.

Norman was soon elected to become a member of the Parochial Church Council. It was necessary as a member of the PCC to attend several meetings a year at which church affairs would be discussed. At each meeting the accounts would be evaluated to enable the church to plan their finances into the future. Ailsa was very appreciative of the fact that the accounts were up to date, as in the past a point had been reached where they were over a year in arrears. Norman did not contribute very much to these discussions and found it difficult to air his views without feeling embarrassed about the relevancy of any comments he might make. The comments and contribution others made during these meetings seemed somehow more relevant than anything he could think of to say. However, the experience of being involved with other people helped reduce his previous awkwardness with others. It made him reassess his own views about his own personality; he no longer regarded himself as being introverted and withdrawn, a description often levied at people with schizophrenia.

One Sunday, Bill made an entrance into the church accompanied by an elderly lady called Jeannie. Bill introduced Norman to her and mentioned that she would like to visit musicals but had no one to accompany her. Norman had probably mentioned to Bill that he enjoyed visiting the theatre but was accustomed to going alone. Jeannie was quite a pleasant person to converse with and had a lot of conversation in her – the type of person Norman felt comfortable with. She seemed lukewarm as far as going out to places was concerned; it seemed to Norman that the idea of trips to the theatre was Bill's. Norman did not feel especially attracted to her physically, although he seemed to relate well with her otherwise. However Norman found her friendly relationship with him quite pleasing. She did have very attractive hair, which she always kept beautifully groomed.

One day Bill confided in Norman that Jeannie had been taken to hospital with a broken hip. Apparently she had experienced a fall in her home, where she had been lying on the floor until Bill had discovered her. Bill had a copy of her flat keys and he was in the habit of visiting her daily. She suffered from epileptic seizures, and apparently had incurred her broken hip while falling down due a seizure. Thankfully, she only had seizures occasionally.

Norman visited her twice in the clinic she had been admitted to, and on one occasion his visit coincided with a friend of Bill's named Ernie, who completely ignored Norman and avoided speaking to him. Norman had encountered Ernie before and it seemed that he was gay. He had been very aggressive to Norman on a previous occasion and had admitted that he had been an athletics coach in the past. He said he had encountered athletes who had been helped financially by Eddie, Norman's bridge partner. According to information on the Internet, Eddie had contributed £2 million to sport. Ernie had made a point that people had insinuated themselves into his favour for monetary advantage. Norman had not been aware that Ernie was gay when he first met him, and Ernie's aggression seemed to Norman due to the fact that Ernie was on the defensive about his sexual orientation.

Bill had suggested to Norman that he should join him in going to the Sunday evening service. Norman concurred and met a black friend of Bill's there called Jim. Jim was a very talkative and humorous person. One Sunday, after the evening service, Jim, Bill, Jeannie and Norman decided to have a drink at the local pub. Norman wasn't very happy about the suggestion as he was not a habitual drinker. However, after a few drinks the conversation came round to Norman's job. Norman confided that he felt he wasn't as popular as he would wish in his place of employment. Bill tactlessly claimed that Norman was paranoid and had an inferiority complex. This remark made Norman feel upset. He felt his relationship with Bill had deteriorated due to that remark and wondered if the accusations levied by Bill were apparent in him to others, if they were indeed true. Norman felt that on some occasions he could have an inflated view of himself and his capabilities, but only lacked confidence.

Norman confided in his mother about the incident and she vehemently said that he was definitely not paranoid. Norman was relieved and believed her as she knew him better than Bill. He had taken Bill into his confidence about a number of personal matters. Bill, however, was to give the impression that he could actually be trusted and Norman wondered if he was letting his imagination run riot about poor Bill, who was kind most of the time. Afterwards, when reflecting on the matter, Norman decided that he might have taken Bill's comments too literally and that he might have overreacted to Bill's wording. Norman had felt disappointed as he had valued Bill as a friend, or at least a close acquaintance.

Norman's journey back home after the evening service with his companions was an opportunity for them all to indulge in trivial conversation after the seriousness of the service just listened to. On the way out of the Lady Chapel there was a print on the wall depicting the Archangel Gabriel announcing to Mary that she is to conceive Jesus, the Saviour of the world. The painting had been executed by Fra Angelico and was appropriate due to the fact that at evening services the Magnificat was always recited. Norman found that his desire to examine such paintings in depth encouraged and deepened his Christian faith. Nearby in the chapel hung a marble bust of the Virgin and Child which continued the story of Mary further.

Norman found the devoutness of most of the congregation something to aspire to himself, although he was very conscious of his own failings. He was more relaxed with the church congregation than the world outside church, but saw that even in church there would be problems with relationships.

Chapter Eighteen – Church Friends

On a later date, Bill asked Norman if he would be interested in accompanying him and Jeannie to a musical event in a local church. Daisy, a regular churchgoer, was present there and was quite convivial, dancing in time to the music during her entrance. After the concert she asked Norman to wait until she returned with an umbrella for him. She had previously been informed that Norman's umbrella had been damaged by a heavy gust of wind. That was the beginning of their relationship and they became friends. She intimated that she was married but the relationship between her and Norman was platonic. She had another friend from church named Ivy, and all three would occasionally go to a restaurant providing jacket potatoes, which Daisy enjoyed. Norman became good friends with Daisy and Ivy, and would socialise with them, although it was Norman's intention that their friendships should be purely platonic.

Ivy's father was confined to bed in a nursing home, as he was in the last stages of Alzheimer's disease. He had to be hand fed and was completely uncommunicative, similar to a baby. She visited him daily and would feed him personally at the appointed time in the evenings. She was very devoted to him and never absented herself from what she regarded as her duty. This made it awkward for Daisy, as she found Ivy's inflexibility a problem when arranging a suitable time for all three of them to go out together. Daisy was easily hurt and would often confide in Norman how upset she was at this person's remark or that person's remark. Norman would try and comfort her, claiming that people were rude to him regularly but that he tried not to dwell on it as that was a part of life.

She had encountered physical problems over the previous few years, having just recovered from a serious kidney problem, which had resulted in her suffering from poor health over a period of two years. She had now recovered and claimed that her prayers for deliverance had been answered, and that it was through her steadfast faith that she overcame her illness. Norman felt an enormous feeling of admiration for her, as she appeared to be a lovely Christian.

Ivy invited Daisy and Norman several times to accompany her on her visits to her father. On one occasion the home provided a birthday celebration for him and all the patients received a share of the cakes. They were all suffering from Alzheimer's disease and some were more communicative than others. Most would respond when spoken to but there were some who were completely locked up in their own world and could not carry out a conversation. One female patient was prompted to indulge in a dance in response to some music and this helped to minimise the serious atmosphere encountered there. Gaiety seemed to replace temporarily the sadness that pervaded the home. Norman realised that despite their difficulty in communicating they were still human beings capable of joy as well as sorrow. Although he tried to stifle the thought, he felt anxious at the possibility of contracting the illness himself in the future. It was brought home to him how important having a sound and healthy mind was to him. His interests all necessitated the application of a keen mind.

Daisy was a very devout Christian and she helped Norman deal with his own spiritual problems. Gertrude's words in response to her son Hamlet's 'constructive' advice to her echoed in Norman's head:

> Thou turnest mine eyes into my very soul,
> And there I see such black and grained spots
> As will not leave their tinct.

Daisy disapproved of his interest in bridge, along with his mother, who disapproved of it as well. Norman disagreed with them and had a conversation with a churchgoer called Caroline, in which he claimed that he was using his mind creatively when playing bridge and that that was using the talents God had given him. After all, he claimed, we are all made in God's image, which includes being creative, just as God is creative. Of course, the degree of creativity a human being normally exhibits is insignificant to that of God.

He was not playing bridge for stakes and was simply playing it for pleasure. He knew some people associated cards with gambling and that they disapproved of cards for this reason. He felt sad that his friend Daisy had this attitude to card playing, although he had derived so much happiness from the game through meeting and interacting with other people who shared his interest in bridge. He felt that playing bridge had improved his skills in interacting with people and had helped him practise building relationships. His mother might have had his best interests at heart in her attitude, and he knew she was proud of his improvement in his human relations.

Ailsa had an assistant priest named Funke who aided her. Funke often addressed Norman as 'Mummy's boy', a comment Norman found distasteful. He tried to analyse her mind and understand why she addressed him in this way. She had noticed him accompanying his mother to the church on some previous occasions and may have assumed that the fact that he was known not to have a close female friend suggested he was over-attached to his mother. Eventually he confronted her about her remarks and asked her bluntly why she often made them. She didn't reply, but from that point onwards she never repeated that phrase again. She had an earthy sense of humour that appealed to Norman. He discovered, from a conversation with her, that she was divorced. Norman realised that his appraisal of the situation might be incorrect, and felt that he might be being oversensitive in imagining that she might have been deliberately unpleasant to him.

She had an attractive daughter called Dami, to whom he had inadvertently betrayed his attraction. Norman would sometimes pay females a compliment on their appearance, but sadly only few responded positively. He was very much aware of the physical beauty of women and felt he had to acknowledge this verbally to them.

Access to the main church was via a long flight of stairs. Some members of the congregation found it difficult to negotiate the stairs as some suffered from mobility problems such as arthritis. Others were unable to climb the stairs at all, and as a result were unable to attend the church. It was therefore decided to raise funds for the purchase and installation of a new lift. This was tackled by holding various activities to raise money for the church and to apply for grants towards the cost of the proposed lift from charities who contributed to good causes such as this.

Norman attended these activities and would often take an active part in the efforts to raise money towards the lift fund. The fund-raising was spread over a period of three years or so. One example was the yearly Vauxhall Park Fair, which the church arranged. On one occasion Norman was in charge of a stall offering a prize for the person who would guess correctly the correct underground station, a winning station having been selected in advance. The winning person was announced over a microphone at the close of the fair. It was Norman's task to make a note of each participant's telephone number in order that they might be contacted in the eventuality of them being successful. Those who participated were mostly very happy and friendly, and Norman felt joy and pleasure at taking part. Once, Joanna Lumley, the actress, had been kind enough to open the fair. Norman was thrilled when he happened to make eye contact with her at the end of the festivities. He occasionally helped in counting the proceeds and depositing it in the bank.

At the meetings of the Parochial Church Council which were held every two months, the progress of the fund-raising was discussed regularly. The up-to-date accounts that Norman provided made it possible for planning from which church funds the money to pay for the lift should be removed. The actual amount required to pay for the lift were reached at the end of three years of effort. This amounted to about £70,000. It was also decided to replace the church hall kitchen, and funds for that purpose were to be removed from the hall fund, which had grown substantially over a number of years, as considerable cash came in from letting the church hall to various organisations on a regular basis.

Ailsa took a leading role in all the activities and remarked that the congregation were leaving a lot of the work to her. The amount required for the lift was eventually raised, the church having had to rely on about £20,000 in grants from various sources. When it was announced that the money had been raised

Norman felt he had, along with many others, achieved something positive and worthwhile.

Chapter Nineteen – Family Crises

Norman's mother and half-brother would visit him every month, coming down from Macclesfield in a hired car. His mother relished the opportunity to be able to see his sister when she visited, as his sister had such an isolated life on her own. She was very concerned about the welfare of his sister while down, and would often shower her with clothes and groceries. Ann would be very grateful and would express her thanks profusely. Norman loved this aspect of Ann's personality and reflected that he should display more gratitude when he himself was offered gifts by his mother. Ann's welfare was very important to Norman as well, as he too loved her. Nora's attitude to Norman seemed to him to be different from that towards his sister, as Norman and his mother would occasionally be involved in unpleasant disagreements. These would often revolve round questions Norman would level at his mother to clarify the discussions they had. He thought she was conscious of her advancing years and did not like to be reminded of this by requests by Norman to clarify her comments. She would also accuse him of being too severe with her. It seemed to Norman that she was being oversensitive to his tone of voice, as she could not accept any firmness on Norman's part. After many years of having disputes their relationship took a turn for the better and the disagreements became much less severe. She claimed that she had prayed as a Christian not to get involved in any further disputes. He wondered if the disagreements had been due to a wrong attitude on his part towards his mother. It was a relief to have overcome that problem they had both faced.

Norman would visit his sister every Sunday. She had to receive regular injections to prevent her from relapsing. As with many others suffering from the same illness, she had to take regular medication for life to avert a possible recurrence of the positive symptoms of schizophrenia. She was not aware of the consequences of discontinuing the injections and it was with horror that one day he noticed that her trousers were torn and her clothes dirty. It seemed she had lost pride in her appearance. Nora was very concerned, and confirmed that she had noticed a change in her behaviour.

Christmas came and Ann, Norman and Nora celebrated it together in his flat. However Ann's behaviour was strange; suddenly she turned on Nora and Norman and made some bizarre accusations against them. The remarks were very distressing to all concerned and it was apparent that she had suffered a relapse. Her clothes were dirty and she looked dishevelled. Eventually she called for a taxi and went home, leaving her mother desperately concerned about her welfare.

Ann was admitted to a mental health clinic. Norman visited her there once a week and found that she had become more subdued due to the treatment she was receiving. He was able to supply her with any necessities she might require in the meantime.

After a period of several weeks she was transferred to a mental hospital. Every week there happened to be a ward round that Norman attended in order to obtain information about how her treatment was progressing, and to be of assistance to those who were medically responsible for her treatment. He was able to give encouraging news about her to her mother, who was very anxious about her condition. Eventually Ann was discharged from hospital and went back to her flat; but even with her cooperation, she never regained the good health she had experienced before this relapse came upon her. It seemed to result in a permanent worsening of her condition, which has remained to this day. She is less communicative and quite withdrawn, making little conversation. Today she often has to be spoken to, as she doesn't as a rule volunteer to take the initiative in conversing with people. She manages her daily basic affairs and looks after herself adequately. She keeps her flat and herself spotlessly clean, and always provides refreshments with generosity when Norman visits her.

One of the ways in which Norman tried to draw Ann out of herself was to make a comment on a plaque hanging on her wall depicting a detail of 'The Swing' by Jean-Honoré Fragonard. This showed a lady dressed in a colourful, frivolous and billowing dress on a swing. A man was partially concealed in the shrubbery with a good vantage point to appreciate the parts of her body that the swinging action exposed. Perhaps Ann was embarrassed by the scene, as she didn't respond much to Norman's efforts at conversation. Norman had experienced tension and discomfort trying to converse with her in the past, but this feeling had been overcome completely in recent years. It was now a joy to be in her presence and he looked forward to his weekly visits to her that he never missed. He hoped that through his efforts in being present regularly for her that her mental condition would improve.

Chapter Twenty – Conclusion

Norman's sister-in-law, Pauline, was his best friend. She was a devout Catholic and was very involved with her own church, having completed a course of studies that she put into good use through instructing beginners in the faith and giving them guidance. Pauline would always greet Norman with a warm and intimate hug and a kiss. She encouraged him in his recreations, including bridge, and that helped to dispel any misgivings he might have had towards it due to criticisms from his mother and Daisy. Pauline realised how important bridge was to him; she appreciated that his relationships at the bridge club helped to improve his personality and allow him to freely interact with people. His psychiatrist had informed him that improving relations with people was a skill that could be learnt, and those words remained in Norman's mind and encouraged him. Pauline's mother was Irish, and was just as sweet and loving to Norman. She also greeted him affectionately by hugging him and kissing him. He felt that physical affection from his own mother was too infrequent. She observed the way he was greeted by Pauline and her mother and commented, 'I never used to receive embraces from my parents when I lived with them. It was something people didn't believe in up there.'

Norman had pondered over the way his mother showed love as compared to the two others, and felt that possibly her love for him was not as deep as she claimed; he had felt something was missing in their relationship. His mother, however, would eventually start to offer her cheek to him to be kissed when they met, so it seemed that she had learned something from the display of affection that Pauline and her mother showed towards him. He was aware that his mother loved him deeply and felt he could have misjudged her attitude, as she showed her love through her kindness and care for him generally.

Norman took over the counting of the offerings and other

income on Sunday mornings in church. They consisted mainly of loose cash, individual envelopes containing money, and cash and cheques from the hire of the church hall. It all had to be entered on an income sheet and banked next day. Bill helped Norman count the offerings and accompanied him to the bank to deposit it into one of the church accounts. The previous people who had been responsible for doing all this had been asked to make way for new people to replace them as they were very elderly and getting a trifle forgetful. Joe, one of them, was reluctant to make way for someone else; he persisted for a while until Ailsa made it clear to him that he was to discontinue that task. Was it Norman's imagination, or did Joe appear disgruntled in church for a period afterwards?

The congregation were encouraged to give 5% of their income to the church, and as the person responsible for the preparation of banking the proceeds from the collection, Norman could see that some were not pulling their weight. It was difficult to ascertain whether a person was giving more or less than what they could afford, as the amounts contributed varied greatly from one person to another. There may well have been among them those who fitted into the category of the poor widow of whom it was said, when she contributed two small coins, 'I tell you the truth, this poor widow has put in more than all the others. All these people gave their gifts out of their wealth; but she out of her poverty put in all she had to live on.'

There was a short regular evening session in church to which about half a dozen elderly members of the congregation came. On the first Sunday of the month there would be held a service of wholeness and healing, which Norman looked forward to; he felt it resulted in an improvement in his mental condition as time went on. Ailsa remarked several times however that there was more to the service than mental or physical healing. She did pronounce the words 'in body, mind and spirit' as she laid hands on those who came forward for healing.

One of those who attended the evening service only was a friend of Bill's called James. He was a very likeable man but admitted that he was not a Christian. When Norman finished work James would suggest they meet at a café on Wednesday afternoons to indulge in a cup of coffee and some toast. Eventually James introduced a Japanese lady called Sati to Norman over the coffee afternoons, and she became a regular attender. However, Norman noticed that James once offered Sati an envelope containing fifty pounds 'for services rendered', which she gratefully accepted.

Norman wondered if there was anything unsavoury about James's relations with Sati.

Norman had approached his practice manager, Helen, to discuss his possible retirement at sixty-five and mentioned that he might retire at retirement age. She advised him to take the decision to retire. As a result, although there was no pressure on Norman to leave, he felt that Helen might be happier if he left. She was replaced by another practice manager, Uma, as Helen had to retire prematurely due to a desire to be with her husband, who was dying of cancer. Helen was a very likeable person and all the staff appreciated her.

On his last day at work it was accidentally revealed to him that there was a party planned for him in the afternoon. Sure enough, he was invited upstairs to the lounge and was amazed to see what could almost be described as a banquet laid out on tables in the lounge! One of the doctors presented him with a cheque for £100 from all four doctors. Norman's colleagues handed him a £50 book token. Other members of staff gave him presents and a card. Norman was very grateful to them, and felt that he had partly at least overcame his personality problems that had made it difficult for him to hold down employment.

Dr Davies, his psychiatrist, had suggested to him to become involved in a patient educator project, where psychiatric patients would conduct mock interviews with trainee doctors in order to give them practical experience in conducting patient interviews. Norman understood that he would receive payment for this, and that the sessions would be one or two hours a week in total. After an initial discussion and one practice session, during which Norman was present to observe how an established patient educator conducted the sessions, he received no further word from the hospital concerned. Norman phoned them several times but was assured that the project was to go ahead. Despite this assurance he was never contacted about the project for the ensuing six months. Afterwards he consoled himself that it was God's will, as possibly it might have been counterproductive to rake over the past week after week with trainee psychiatrists or doctors.

Norman had been fortunate enough in his relations with people at the bridge club to have exchanged phone numbers with about a dozen people who would occasionally phone him to arrange to play with him. One lady, Jennifer, arranged to play with him regularly on Tuesdays. She was in the process of separating from her husband, and confessed she had suffered from mental health problems. She invited him and two lady members of the bridge club to a bridge evening at her apartment. She was kind enough to supply a three course meal for all her guests. She mentioned that she possessed a painting valued at £60,000, and shared Norman's interest in art. However, after some subsequent disastrous results playing bridge with her, she suggested they dissolve their partnership, as she felt she was letting him down.

He met an elderly Asian lady at the club called Rajani. They shared a common interest in Bollywood movies, Norman admitting that he had about fifty Bollywood DVDs. They seemed to get on well together and arranged to play regularly. However Norman felt she was slightly critical of his bidding and play, and like many was oblivious to her own mistakes. However, the partnership continued and she seemed quite happy for it to remain so.

Eventually Norman received word from the hospital that they would be resuming the training for those who wished to be involved in the patient educator project. During one practice session in the presence of some other aspiring patient educators, Norman was 'interviewed' by a medical student, to whom he was frank about his sexual experiences. At the end of the training she expressed her disapproval briefly but was admonished by the lecturer in communications who was present. By and large, however, he found that the reactions of the others were favourable; he ended up feeling that he might have been hypersensitive in the past about these matters. He was able to start his part-time work as a patient educator and quite enjoyed the experience.

Looking back on his past, Norman felt he had made great strides in overcoming his emotional problems and his illness of schizophrenia. It seemed practically inconceivable to him that he would have any more relapses, as he had become more hardened to other people's brusqueness and rudeness, factors that had contributed towards his previous relapses. His medication was very effective as well, and he had no pronounced side effects from it. In addition, his Christian life was extremely important to him, and it had been suggested to him by Ailsa that he should study for a certificate in theology, a challenge he accepted. He had some friends, and things could only improve in the future. He had never fallen in love but was assured of the love of Christ towards him and he was content with that.

He spent a considerable amount of time reading his notes on each course lecture and the course was instrumental in helping him focus on the Bible. He would research his assignments enthusiastically and apply himself diligently to the course. His involvement in his church and his friends there went some way towards healing the scars that had been inflicted on his mind in the past. He hoped to improve his concentration in church when listening to the sermon, and joined in enthusiastically with the hymn singing. He prayed regularly and found that this made Jesus more real and close to him. His Christian faith was the most important thing in his life, and it had been pivotal towards his recovery from schizophrenia. As a result, he knew he could face the future with confidence, remembering the words of Paul in Philippians 3:13–14:

> Forgetting what is behind and straining toward what is ahead, I press on toward the goal to win the prize for which God has called me heavenward in Christ Jesus.

Amen.

Contacts

www.schizophrenia.com

www.healthline.com

Mind – www.mind.org.uk

Mental Health Foundation – www.mentalhealth.org.uk

NIHME
Wellington House
Area 226
133–155 Waterloo Road
London
SE1 8UG

Mental Health Matters,
Avalon House
St. Catherine's Court
Sunderland Enterprise Park
Sunderland
SR5 3XJ

Sane,
1st Floor,
Cityside House,
40 Adler Street,
London,
E1 1EE

LaVergne, TN USA
20 January 2010
170664LV00001B/25/P